Pilates | Personal Trainer

POWERHOUSE **Abs** WORKOUT

Pilates | Personal Trainer

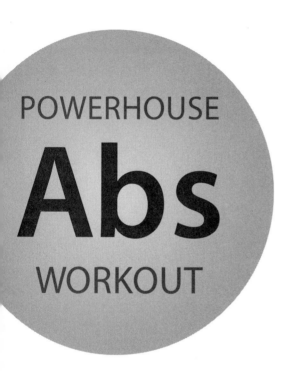

POWERHOUSE

Abs

WORKOUT

Illustrated step-by-step matwork routine

Michael King

Yolande Green

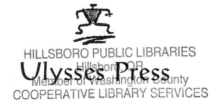

Ulysses Press

Published in the United States by
Ulysses Press
P.O. Box 3440
Berkeley, CA 94703
www.ulyssespress.com

Published in the United Kingdom as *Pilates: The Complete Body
System* (2002) and *Pure Pilates* (2000) by Mitchell Beazley, an
imprint of Octopus Publishing Group Ltd

Library of Congress Card Number 2002105373
ISBN 1-56975-322-9

3/22/1996   9/04

Printed in Canada by Transcontinental Printing

10 9 8 7 6 5 4 3 2 1

Interior Design	Kenny Grant
Cover Design	Sarah Levin
Photography	Ruth Jenkinson
Models	Beth Caterer
	Nancy Markwick
	Malcolm Muirhead
	Simon Spalding

Distributed in the United States by Publishers Group West
and in Canada by Raincoast Books

Please Note
This book has been written and published strictly for informational
purposes, and in no way should be used as a substitute for
consultation with health care professionals. You should not
consider educational material herein to be the practice of medicine
or to replace consultation with a physician or other medical
practitioner. The author and publisher are providing you with
information in this work so that you can have the knowledge and
can choose, at your own risk, to act on that knowledge. The
author and publisher also urge all readers to be aware of their
health status and to consult health care professionals before
beginning any health program.

contents

INTRODUCTION

VITAL ELEMENTS

THE WORKOUT

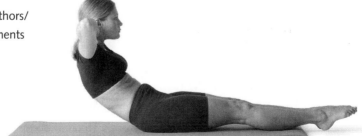

introduction

Pilates is not a fitness fad; it is a holistic concept that will not only make you feel fitter and more flexible, but will enrich your whole way of life. The series of movements will not only change how your body looks, but it will also give you a new physical poise and greater mental strength.

During my years as an exercise instructor, I have witnessed many trend shifts in the fitness industry—from high impact to low impact aerobics, from slide to step, and from spinning to core and functional training. Some of these changes have been introduced because of safety concerns over certain movements or ways of exercising. The advantage of a Pilates system, in contrast, is that the movements can be gentle on your body. The technique can also be effectively used to complement other exercise regimes.

I am one of a third generation of Pilates instructors following Joseph Pilates and writing this book is part of my effort to give others an insight into the power of the Pilates way. I would like to pass on all the information and knowledge that I have developed over my years in the fitness industry, training people in the physical skills to enrich the quality of their lives.

It is very exciting to witness the current popularity of Pilates. From the perspective of someone with a back injury who has worked with many different types of exercise, I have seen the value of the Pilates technique and the way that it changes people. You may believe that a hunched posture is part of getting older, but this is not the case. If you pay regular attention to your body and invest in it by incorporating stretching and challenging exercises into your routines, then you will benefit by feeling fitter and more attractive. You can also maintain these benefits as you grow older.

Balancing your body

Pilates is a system of exercise that, when regularly practiced, will improve your flexibility and strength. The movements will have a noticeable impact on your body in terms of general well-being, youthfulness, and flexibility, and they will also help to heal any long-

or short-term injuries. Even moderate regular daily activities may result in recurring aches or physical problems. Sitting at a desk all day, for example, unbalances your body, causing the hip flexors (the front muscles of your thighs) and the upper back to form themselves into a rounded position. Pilates helps to release such tensions and ease your body back into a more natural balance. It also helps you to achieve a leaner body, feel more poised, less anxious, and stronger mentally. The moves shown here are structured with this in mind and are based on the movements that Joseph Pilates taught.

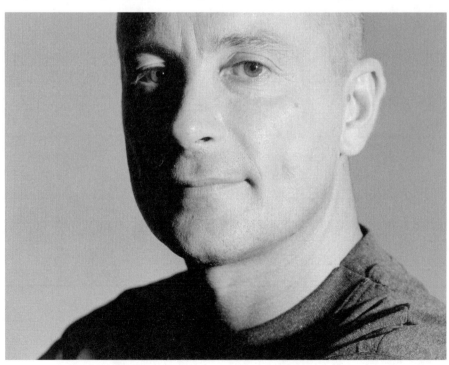

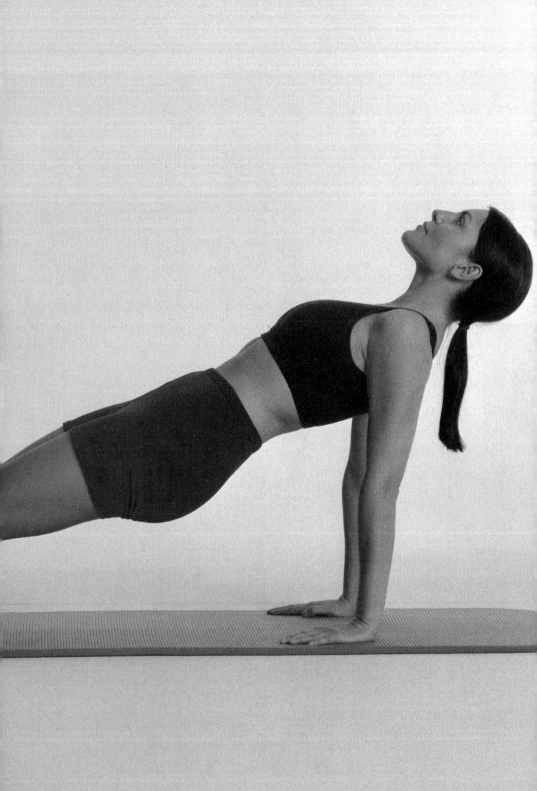

why Pilates?

The Pilates movements stretch the muscles and pull them into a longer and leaner shape, rather than forcing them to tear and rebuild into the shorter and thicker shape that conventional strength training does.

Pilates systematically exercises all the muscle groups in your body, challenging the weak areas as well as the strong. It balances the body, focuses on tight areas, and aims to increase strength and flexibility. When he conceived the original matwork exercises, Joseph Pilates was looking to stretch the body to the full to bring maximum benefit to the person exercising. Even experienced athletes may find some of his original moves difficult. This is because they use muscle control and coordination that few people are used to.

All-round benefits

The Pilates system works the body as a whole, and aims to coordinate the upper and lower muscle groups with the center of the body. This has a dramatic effect on strength, flexibility, posture, and coordination. Whether you are interested in Pilates for cosmetic, medical, or preventative reasons, the system of movements will strengthen your body and at the same time focus your mind.

Anyone can do it

You do not have to be an athlete to be involved with Pilates. And while the exercises are designed to put a minimum of strain on the body, they also aim to challenge its capabilities. This means that anyone of any age and any level of fitness can do Pilates. Whether young or old, a fitness fanatic or someone who has never exercised before, you will reap the benefits.

Basic equipment

You don't need any expensive equipment for Pilates exercises; you can follow a program at home with just a floor mat. The Pilates system is often linked to various innovative Pilates machines, equipment that can form an integral part of the exercises. However, remember that there is nothing that you can do on a machine that you can't do on the mat.

Develops concentration

Known as the intelligent way of working out, there is a focus on concentration and discipline with Pilates. Standard exercise regimes tend not to require mental discipline, but Pilates is different, healing and treating the mind and body on different levels. And because it works all the muscles in the body, simple everyday tasks such as shopping or gardening also become easier and safer.

Pilates and yoga

Pilates and Yoga have certain goals in common. Most significantly they both advocate individual progress in a non-competitive format. The exercises also share an emphasis on stretching, as well as strengthening muscles. Both Yoga and Pilates emphasize deep breathing and the use of smooth, long movements that encourage muscles to relax and lengthen. Pilates is also similar to Yoga because of the body suppleness it brings. The difference is that while some Yoga techniques involve moving from one static posture to the next without repetitions, Pilates flows through a series of movements that are more dynamic, systematic, and anatomically based.

Popular support

Although Pilates has been around since the 1920s, an understanding of this program of exercise that builds up your strength and your immune system has only become popular quite recently. Many Hollywood stars have endorsed the technique—among them Sharon Stone, Courtney Cox Arquette, Minnie Driver, Julia Roberts, and Madonna (who has even claimed that it is the only way to exercise). As a result, Pilates is no longer the domain of the rich and famous and can be practiced in most gyms and health clubs.

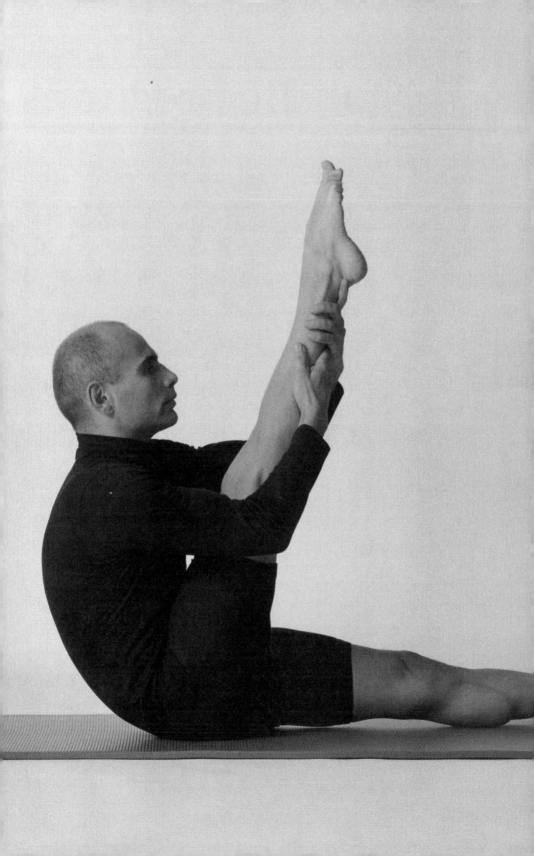

holistic program

Pilates is a thinking way of moving, and involves making a serious commitment to your body and your well-being. It is not an exercise regime to be compartmentalized in your life.

Pilates is significantly more effective when combined with enough restful sleep, a healthy diet, and a complementary fitness program. So Pilates is an invaluable, solid support system for any other regular exercise that you are involved in. It is now accepted that various fitness regimes, such as aerobics, swimming, gym work, or bodybuilding—are not inappropriate, but simply insufficient. An unbalanced exercise regime will not prepare the body for every eventuality. Even though injuries are limited in exercise classes or gyms because of thorough warming-up techniques and health-and-safety regulations, it is still common to pull muscles when lifting heavy items at home or work. What we need to adopt, and what Pilates offers, is a way of training the different parts of the body to work together, to support each other and give your body the protection that it needs.

Cross-training

Just because you have started to exercise using the Pilates method, it does not mean that you have to give up on other sports and fitness programs. On the contrary, your Pilates program is best served when it is complemented by a form of cardiovascular exercise. Complete low-stress Pilates exercises alongside aerobic ones. You will find Pilates ideal for cross-training because it will correct any postural problem associated with other forms of repetitive exercise. Pilates embraces all the areas that make up a fully integrated approach to fitness: strength, flexibility, motor skills, coordination, and relaxation.

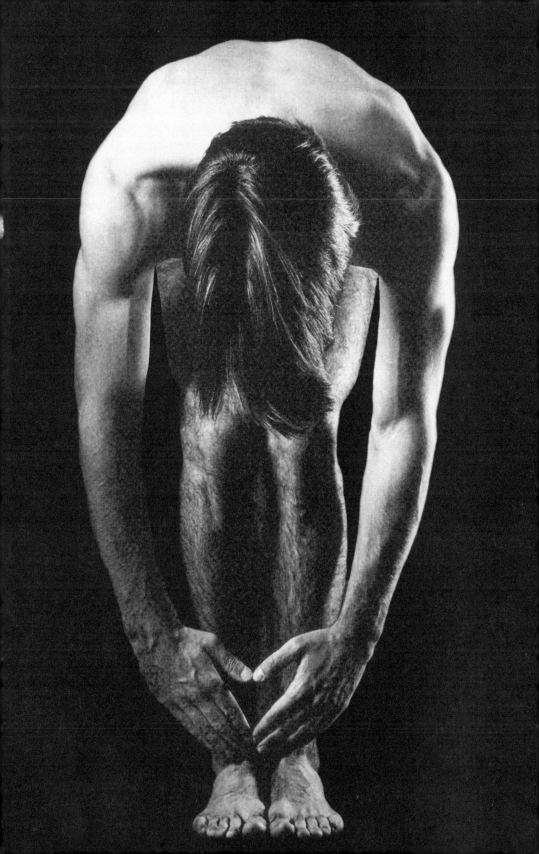

the workout

What would you like to gain from this workout? You will need to understand where your physical strengths and weaknesses lie in order to focus on exercises that will benefit you most.

Weaknesses do not only signify a lack of muscular strength, but also relate to tight areas of your body that hold you back from fully performing a task. Remember, an inflexible body will result in the same problems as one with no muscular strength.

You will find that the exercises you least enjoy are generally those your body needs to spend more time on. In the same way, those that are easier will need to be practiced less.

The workout in this book is in no way meant to replace your holistic fitness program, nor substitute for a general Pilates regimen. I have designed this focused abdominal workout as a supplemental workout to address your weakness in this one area. When added to your regular workout program, it can help bring your body into better balance.

Pure Pilates

Joseph Pilates' original book featured a series of 34 movements. I present many of these pure Pilates exercises, along with beginner variations of the moves, in my book *Pilates Workbook*. Although I would like all my students to be able to undertake the full range of these movements, as a responsible fitness leader I need to work around their capabilities.

Joseph Pilates developed his technique from instinct, and although the basic principles always remained the same, when he worked with particular students he adapted the moves according to their requirements.

So, an essential part of Pilates is knowing what you *cannot* do.

Always listen to your body, both when exercising and once you have finished, and be sensitive to any vulnerable areas.

Pacing yourself

Undertaking advanced moves at the beginning of a Pilates program is unwise. The original Pilates moves are advanced and inappropriate for those unfamiliar with the correct techniques. If you challenge yourself with Pilates exercises that are beyond your level or are uncomfortable, you then risk possible injury. If you stay sensitively attuned to your body and gradually challenge yourself, you can then move toward your ultimate goals at an effective pace.

Note: The moves in this book are at an intermediate to advanced level.

Challenge yourself

Remember that over the long run you should exercise equally across the full range of body movements rather than concentrating on particular movements and specific muscle groups. However, if you are weak in the abdominal area, you need to challenge yourself more in this region. This is important in order to rebalance your body and enable it to perform the more demanding Pilates movements.

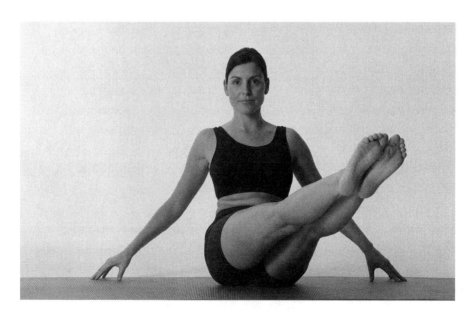

preventing pain

Even the most healthy person may have minor pains that indicate stresses and strains on the body. Never ignore these symptoms, but use them to identify which areas need more strengthening or more stretching and mobility.

Pilates trains the body to prevent injury and to maintain good posture and movement. In order to have good posture, you need to develop good muscle balance. Indeed, injuries are often related in some way to bad posture or muscular imbalances. These types of problems can occur for many reasons. Repetitive movements can be one cause, such as when a golfer continuously practices his swing on one side of the body or when someone spends long periods of time working at a desk. In fact, any pattern that destabilizes your body's natural balance and makes it tense, can lead to weakness, tightness, and a resulting danger of injury.

Pain and Gain

There is always a certain amount of discomfort that arises during training, especially when it comes to stretching muscles that you may not have used in some time. A strong stretch may elicit some pain, but be careful not to push yourself too far. If any pain is sudden or sharp you must stop immediately. This extreme should never be experienced. I emphasize again that Pilates should be performed gradually. It is always better to build up slowly. Only in this way can you strike a balance between achievement and challenge. Never exercise when you are in chronic pain or when any of your muscles are inflamed.

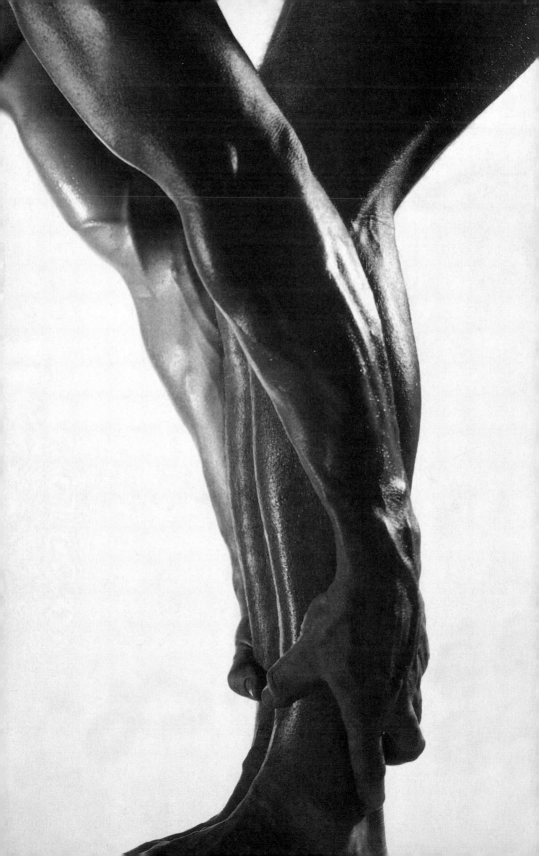

vital elements

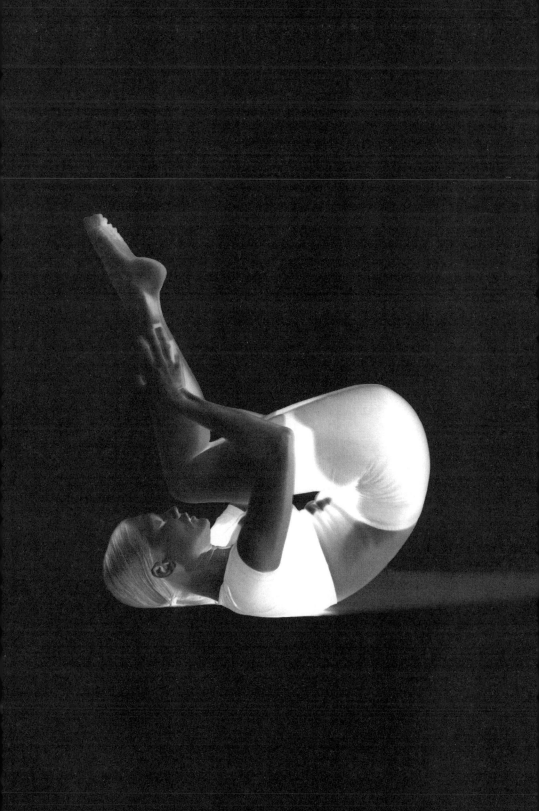

concentration

With many exercise classes and techniques you don't have to think about what you're doing, you just do it to get through it. But with Pilates, every movement is a conscious act controlled by the power of your mind.

"Always keep your mind wholly concentrated on the purpose of the exercises as you perform them." Joseph Pilates

Pilates is "the thinking way of moving" and requires a different kind of concentration than that typically used for other exercise forms. It may not be all that important to concentrate during an aerobics class or when walking on a treadmill, but it is absolutely essential for Pilates.

Setting the mood

There are simple things you can do to improve concentration. Check that the space you plan to use for Pilates is free of distractions and that it is warm and comfortable. Make sure you will not be disturbed.

Though Pilates is not a spiritual workout, you will find it very relaxing because concentrating on a single movement causes everything else that is going on in your life to fade away.

If you want to use music in the background, make sure it isn't punctuated by a heavy beat. Don't make the mistake I once made

Controlling our thoughts, much like controlling our actions, is not as easy as it might first appear to be. When you are under pressure, your thoughts can become very erratic and spin off in random directions. If you are stressed, going to sleep can be especially difficult because you are unable to "switch off." Unwelcome thoughts pop into your head despite your best efforts.

Effective concentration is a skill we acquire as children. By the time we are adults, we all have a little "inner voice" that controls our actions.

First attempts at unfamiliar movements may feel strange and awkward. It is very easy to fall into the trap of performing only the moves you enjoy, when what you need most is to do the ones you do not like. Normally people speed up the difficult part of the movement to get it over with as soon as they can. Instead, you need to slow down. Only by concentrating on what you are doing can you properly control your actions.

when I used a tape of nature sounds that featured screeching parrots and mating whales!

A clear mind

You'll soon find that the benefits of practicing concentration—easier mental focus, clarity of thought, and, most importantly, reduction of stress—are well worth the effort.

All too often in our whirlwind modern lives visual clutter and noisy distractions make it difficult to focus on the task at hand. Stress itself makes concentration more difficult but persevere; mental focus is an art that improves with practice. Marshalling your powers of concentration helps you feel calmer and in control.

Making time for Pilates

Because concentration is linked to focusing on priorities, it is also needed when you are planning your exercises. Start with small sessions of 20–30 minutes, and aim to work up to an hour. It is better to have 20 minutes of a rewarding workout than an hour simply going through the motions of a routine.

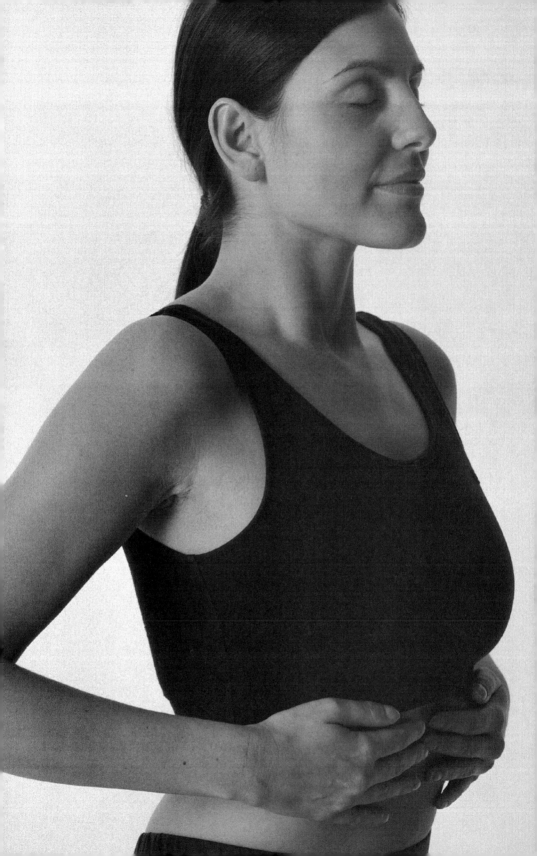

breathing

Pilates uses a controlled and continuous way of breathing that takes time to perfect, but results in a stronger and more energy-efficient body.

"Breathing is the first act of life. Our very life depends on it. Millions have never learned to master the art of correct breathing."

Joseph Pilates

As babies and young children, we breathe correctly, but as adults we tend to develop poor breathing patterns. Correct breathing ensures a good flow of oxygen to the working muscles, which then cleanses the bloodstream and energizes the whole body. Breathing also improves concentration and aids smooth and fluid movement.

There are many types of breathing techniques, and different types can make movements easier, harder, or more controlled. A correct breathing technique can be mastered, but it takes time and patience.

So how should we breathe?

In Pilates, we follow a breath called thoracic or lateral breathing. This means breathing wide and full into your back and sides, opening the ribcage as you breathe. Think of your lungs as bellows, expanding and widening as you breathe in and closing down as you breathe out. This way of breathing works the intercostal muscles, the muscles between the ribs. When these muscles are working, the upper body is more mobile and fluid in its movements.

Pilates exercises are designed in combination with breathing techniques to work the correct muscles to create the required movement. The core muscles always support this process.

Normal breathing

When you inhale normally, the lungs expand, the diaphragm drops and the stomach moves out. As you exhale, your diaphragm lifts and the stomach moves in. This is called "abdominal" breathing and is quite natural.

The wrong way

Whatever you do, don't hold your breath. Most people hold their breath if they pick up something heavy, much as weightlifters would when picking up a barbell. This type of breathing is called the Valsalvic method and results in a stressful increase in blood pressure. It wastes energy in parts of the body where it isn't required. In Pilates you want to keep your breathing continuous.

Muscles that make up the core

The following groups of muscles make up your core or center.
- *TA (transverse abdominal) muscles* are the corset-like muscles that wrap around the center of your body.
- *Multifidus muscles* run down the length of the spine. They link two or three vertebrae and can create or block movement.
- *The pelvic floor* is the sling muscle that runs from the front of the pelvis to the lower part of the spine.
- *The diaphragm* is the muscle that lies under the ribcage and helps you to inhale and exhale.

Thoracic breathing exercise

Sit comfortably or stand tall. Place your hands on the front of your ribcage with your fingertips just touching. As you breathe in, fill the lungs, open the ribcage, and let the fingers slide apart. As you breathe out, let them slide back to touch again. This can take considerable practice. To advance the exercise, move your hands farther around so that your hands are touching your armpits, and breathe to push your ribcage into your hands. If you can reach, extend your palms around to your back.

Another option is to place both hands on the front of the ribcage and breathe first into the right hand, then into the left hand, then into both hands equally. This will increase your body awareness and your breathing control.

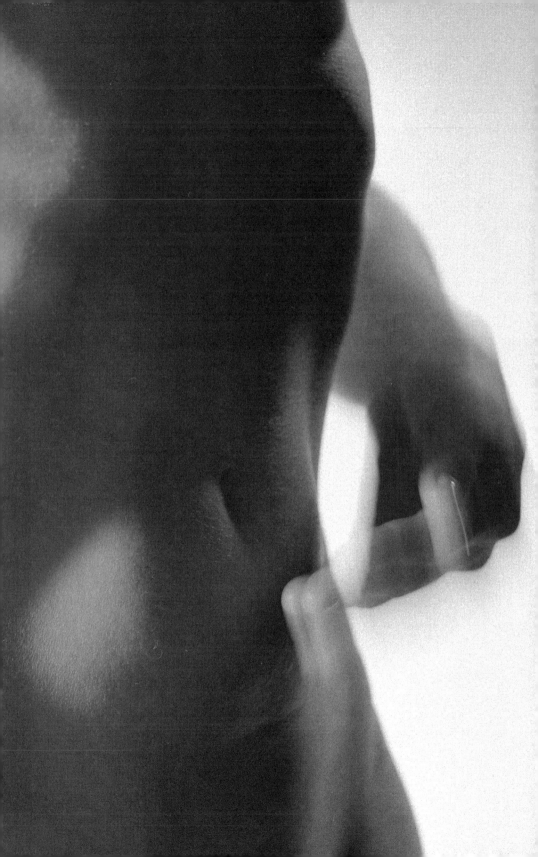

centering

The body is designed to work as a complete unit. If you train to do this, you will have a solid center to create the physical power for each movement. In order to visualize the body as an integrated unit, think of a conductor bringing together all the sections of an orchestra to perform a concerto.

Joseph Pilates believed that our abdominal muscles, now known as abs, function as the "powerhouse" for the whole of the body. Your abs are your center and they initiate every movement. To maintain a strong center you need an equal balance of strength between the abs and the back.

The core

We have already referred to the core (see breathing on page 23) as consisting of four muscle groups: the TA muscles, the multifidus muscles (back muscles), the pelvic floor muscles, and the diaphragm.

Imagine your core as a tree trunk, the core being the solid supporting center of your arms, legs, and head. If you imagine cutting through the tree trunk, the muscles of your body represent the rings of age in the tree: The global muscles (the rectus abdominus muscle) are on the outside of the trunk. As you move toward the center you'll find the external oblique muscles, the internal oblique muscles, and finally the TA muscles.

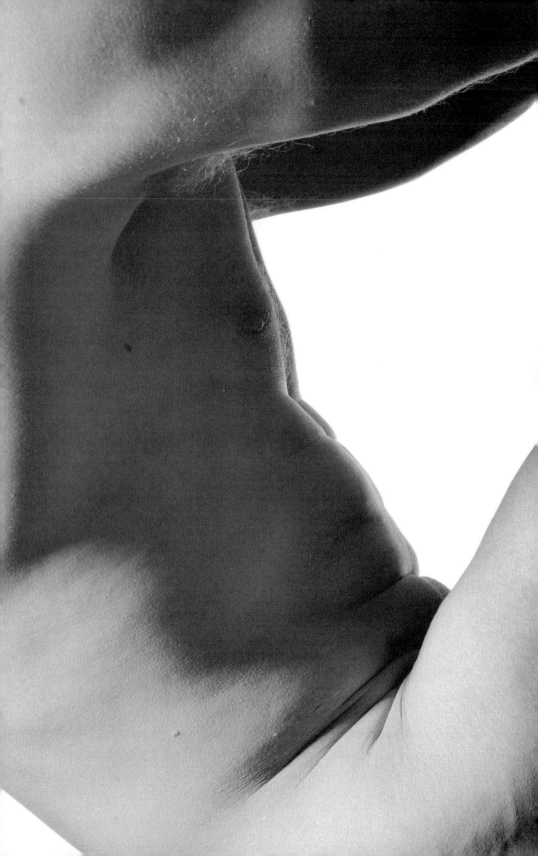

30 percent contraction

Every exercise is controlled or initiated from the contraction of two of the core muscles, the TA muscles or the pelvic floor. This is because these muscles help to stabilize the body as you move.

For many years, Pilates practitioners would pull in the lower abdominal muscles tighter as the movement became more challenging. Now, however, research has established that this is not the most effective way to work these muscles. Drawing in the abdominal muscles as hard as you can activates the core muscles with what I call 100 percent effort. This tires the muscles quickly, and it does not train them to operate effectively in everyday activities. Research has shown that the most effective way to train them is at 30 percent of their maximum strength. This allows them to be used throughout an hour's session without causing fatigue. They will also become naturally stronger and support you as you perform your daily activities. Work through the following exercises to help you to find your center.

Pelvic floor and TA muscles

Activate your center either through the TA muscles (shown opposite) or by using the pelvic floor muscles. Research has shown that it is not productive to use both muscles together, so when following your routine, try to activate your center by using only one group of muscles.

Activating the TA muscles

Imagine that you have a belt around your waist and that the abdominal muscles draw in when you tighten it. Use the images on page 29 (stages 1–3) to establish the most efficient level at which to perform the exercises.

Activating the pelvic floor

The pelvic floor runs from the front of the pelvis to the lower spine and supports you like a sling. This is one of the hardest muscles to activate, but when mastered it will be easy to practice wherever you are without anyone knowing. You can activate the pelvic floor muscle by imagining that you are trying to stop your urine in mid-flow.

Imagine that your pelvic floor is the floor of an elevator. As you breathe out, draw up the elevator as far as you can to the tenth floor. Then release this halfway to the fifth floor and then a little farther to the third floor. This is the level of exertion that you want to follow in the program. Continue the exercise with the following pattern: move the elevator to the tenth floor, return to the ground floor, up again to the fifth floor, and back to the ground floor. Finally go up to the third floor and back down. When you do this exercise, you can be sitting or standing—the key is to be comfortable.

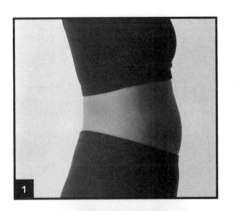

1 In a standing position, allow your abdominal muscles to relax and form a dome. Don't push them out. Instead, become aware of how the rest of your body feels as you release these muscles.

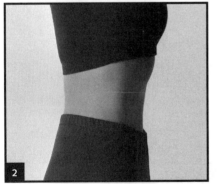

2 As you breathe out, draw in the abdominal muscles as far as you can. Imagine that a belt is being tightened around you, that it will be tightened right up to the last notch. This is what I call 100 percent effort.

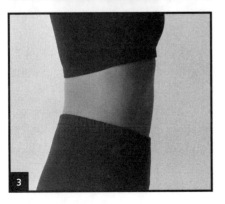

3 Relax the muscles halfway to reach the "fifth notch" on the belt. Think of this as 50 percent effort. Then release them a little more to the "third notch," or 30 percent effort. This is the level at which to work efficiently throughout your program.

VITAL ELEMENTS

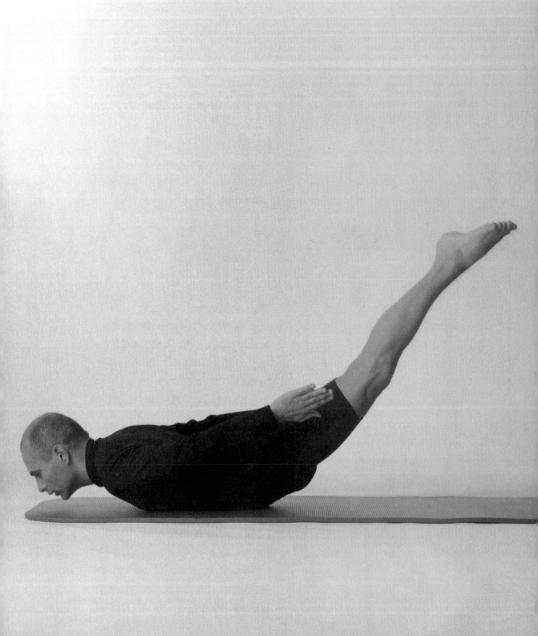

control

Good posture can be achieved only when the body is under perfect control. When doing the exercises, aim for slow, studied movements, and allow them to flow from start to finish to form a continuous sequence. Continue in this way until you have completed the total number of repetitions.

Working with the weight of your body against the natural pull of gravity requires considerable control. In fact, we are all accustomed to controlling our bodies: the process of walking is not a haphazard series of movements, but rather a controlled sequence that we have learned from childhood. However, many of us, quite unconsciously, developed bad habits in the way that we move that may later affect our physical health.

Maintaining control means ensuring that the body moves with purpose and direction at all times. A controlled movement involves making the relevant muscles and joints work to their full capacity while at the same time not wasting any energy. This concept is integral to the philosophy of Pilates.

Pilates exercises strengthen the body, and the slower and more controlled the movements, the greater the strength you gain from them.

Visualization

The use of visual associations can be effective when working with

Pilates. Visualization can help you understand how to control your movements and also how to gain the most from your workouts.

For example, I have already noted that Pilates exercises need to be continuous, to flow from one stage to another freely, without interruption. So, if you are trying a new movement, it might be helpful to think, as you begin, of a Ferris wheel at a fairground—the wheel turning slowly and deliberately. Or, think of a tightrope walker at the circus. In order to stay on the rope she has to maintain perfect control of her body, to move slowly and deliberately from one end of the rope to the other. Such visualizations are used throughout this book to give you deeper insight into how each exercise should feel.

The powerhouse

In disciplines such as tai chi, it is believed that the powerhouse is the store of the *chi*, or life energy. With physical movements, the energy is generated from the powerhouse, then carried to the relevant part of the body to give it power. This is equivalent to the core or center in Pilates.

Graceful control

When practicing Pilates, make every movement as smooth and graceful as you can. To use a visualization, imagine that you are a dancer performing a movement on a stage in front of an audience you want to impress with your grace and poise.

Think, too, about every part of your body as you move. Does each part have an important role in the execution of the movement, and are both sides of your body

VITAL ELEMENTS

Resist me

Find a partner. Stand up, holding a towel in your right hand. Have your partner sit down at your feet and hold the other end of the towel with both hands. Pull your fist, with the towel, toward your shoulder in a bicep curl. Let your partner create resistance so that there is equal tension as you move your arm up and down.

Think about a resistance scale from one to ten. One is when your partner exerts no resistance with the towel. Ten is when your partner pulls so hard that you can't move at all. Aim for a resistance level of five in both directions. Breathe out as you curl the arm up and breathe in as you uncurl the muscle. Repeat 10 times and change arms.

Next, drop the towel but imagine you are still holding it and repeat the bicep curl. Do you feel the resistance that you had when you were holding the towel? This technique will aid controlled action.

Slower is harder

Begin by doing five regular push-ups, either with your legs fully extended in the full push-up position, or with your knees on the floor (the three-quarter position). Do these first five at your normal pace.

Now do another five, but count two slow counts down and two slow counts up. Breathe in as you go down and out as you come up. Rest. Now repeat, but to a count of four in each direction. Rest. Finally, try a last five push-ups, to a count of six on the way down and another six on the way up, without pausing at the top or at the bottom, making all five push-ups one long, continuous, and steady movement. It was harder than you thought, wasn't it?

At this latter point you are working at the same intensity that you should be working at while doing the Pilates exercises. Pilates is all about quality and range of movement, with the contraction of the muscles (the downward movement in this case) and the flexion (the pushing up movement) requiring equal effort.

steady, and even movements. You will be able to feel the difference and the exercises will prove more effective (you may have to use a lighter weight).

It is also vitally important to ensure that you are using your full range of movement. Check that you are working equally hard, with the same intensity and resistance throughout. As much effort should be used to extend a muscle (eccentric movement) as to contract it (concentric movement). By working in this way, you will begin to develop strength and flexibility in equal measure, giving your muscles (and your body) a long, lean look.

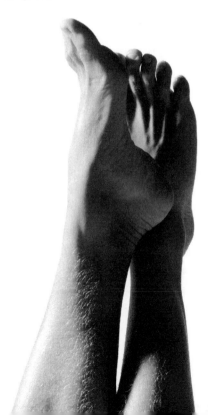

working at the same level? If not, rebalance yourself so that each part has an equal role.

Full range

This type of movement can be applied to other forms of exercise with much success: try using resistance machines or free weights in the gym with slow,

posture

Good posture is vital. Having bad posture will prevent your body from functioning efficiently, and it will also undermine your balance and coordination. The danger is that if you develop a habit of having bad posture, your body will accept it as normal and will learn to suffer any associated aches and pains.

An ideal posture will have all the joints in a neutral position so that they are without stress. The joint will follow the natural alignment of the bones. A neutral position will reduce wear on the joints, promote balance, and keep the muscles around the joints in correct alignment. This in turn allows the internal organs to feel comfortable and function efficiently. It is important that you establish a neutral position before you start each exercise.

Poor posture

Poor posture can lead to many adverse symptoms, which include:

- *Fatigue*
- *Neck and shoulder tension*
- *Headaches*
- *Impaired balance and coordination*
- *Muscular weakness*
- *Poor circulation*
- *Tension and stress*
- *Digestive problems*
- *Aching and painful joints*

Correcting poor posture

There are the three main types of problematic posture: sway-back (see stage 1), lordosis (see stage 2), and kyphosis (rounding of the shoulders or hunching). It is also possible to have a combination of these postures.

Poor posture can be corrected, but it will take time and patience. As well as realignment exercises, you will need to give your body time to adjust to a different position. Some bad postures can be corrected surprisingly quickly while others need more time to fix.

The plumbline test

Assess your posture in front of a full-length mirror, wearing just your underwear. Stand in profile, and turn your head to the mirror.

Imagine a plumbline hanging from your ear and look at the joints that the line runs through. With a healthy posture, the line should run through the ear lobe, the center of the neck, the tip of the shoulder, the center of the ribcage, slightly behind the hip joint, the center of the knee joint, and just in front of the anklebone.

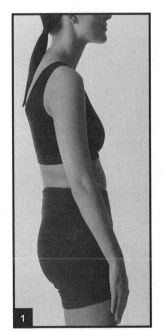 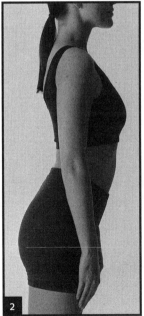 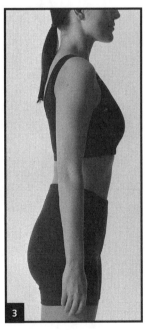

1 Sway-back posture, often called the slouch position, is common among teenagers.

2 The lordotic posture is characterized by an increased curve in the lower part of the spine.

3 With an ideal posture, gravity is evenly distributed and all joints are in their neutral position.

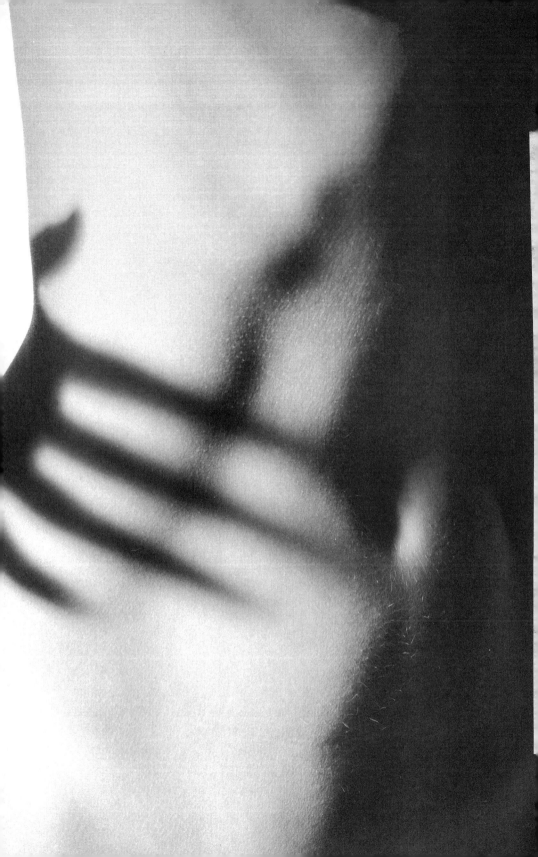

neutral spine

A neutral spine is used to describe when your spine is in its most natural position. This will not necessarily be the position that feels most comfortable. It is quite likely that your "normal" posture has been created by poor habits and you have become accustomed to the way it feels.

Finding a position with a neutral spine can be a real challenge. It is essential, however, that you find your neutral position and sustain it before undertaking any Pilates moves. Once you have started the exercises that follow, you will need to learn to hold the neutral position as your body is moving.

Training out of neutral

If your body loses the correct neutral position as you exercise the benefit to you is lost. In this scenario, you are simply making your body stronger in your preferred, non-neutral position, one that has been created by bad habits. Training in a non-neutral position also increases your chances of acquiring muscular imbalances, injuries, and increasing tension because your body is not adequately supported.

Pelvis and spine

While it is important that *all* your joints are in neutral during the moves, this section focuses on the pelvis and spine. The position of the pelvis and the position of the lower spine always affect each other. If your pelvis is rolled forward, for example, the curve in your lower spine will be exaggerated, and will not form a neutral position.

Finding neutral

You should always practice finding neutral either by lying down or by standing—the principle is the same—before starting any exercises. Most people find that lying down is the easier way to start because the floor provides some support. Follow the stages described below to find neutral.

Stage one

This stage shows the spine out of neutral with an increased lower spine curve. Start by lying on the floor in a relaxed position with your knees bent and your feet flat on the floor. Softly tilt the pelvis forward so that the space under your lower back increases. Be careful not to push this position too far because it may cause discomfort in your lower spine. See how each part of your body—particularly your legs, chest, and arms—feels in this position. Then relax back out of the position.

Stage two

The second picture shows the spine out of neutral with no lower spine curve. In the same lying position, softly tilt your pelvis back

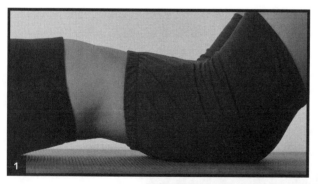

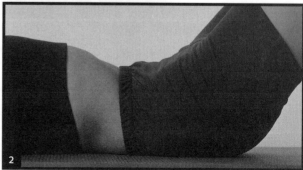

and visualize imprinting your lower spine into the mat. Don't push this position too far, and stop if it feels uncomfortable. Notice how each part of your body—particularly your legs, abdominal muscles, back, and waist—feels in this position. Then relax back out of the position.

Stage three

The third picture shows the spine in neutral. To find this position, shift your body between stages one and two, and find a position halfway between the two points. This should leave a small space under your lower back. Notice how each part of your body feels in this position—there should be no tension in the legs, chest, or back.

Stage four

The fourth stage shows the clock technique, another way to help find neutral.

Place your hands on your lower abdominal muscles with your little fingers pointing down toward your pubic bone. Imagine that your hands are a clockface (with the fingers pointing to 12 o'clock and your thumbs pointing to 6 o'clock). Tilt the pelvis forward and backward, so that 12 o'clock is higher, then 6 o'clock is higher. Neutral is the position where 12 o'clock and 6 o'clock are level.

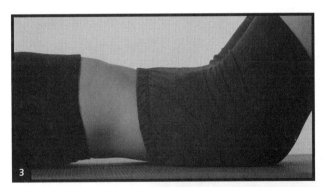

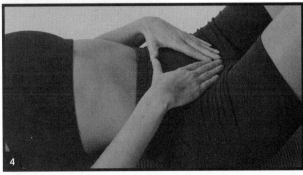

precision

You have your own natural geometry. Pilates can help you move with more precision and discover for yourself the dimensions of natural grace.

All Pilates movements are exact, and involve precise actions and precise breathing. When you think of precision and movement, you might think of synchronized swimmers or the exacting choreography that dancers can achieve. Joseph Pilates trained as both a boxer and an acrobatic circus performer, which gave him an appreciation of precision skills as well as an acute awareness of space and time.

Perfect reach

Bring to mind the image of the spread-eagled figure drawn by Leonardo da Vinci. The artist drew a circle around the figure as he stretched out to his fullest extent. These lines of geometry are a useful visualization of the space around us. Or, imagine the arm of a ballet dancer arching like the tip of a compass; we are all capable of making similar pin points in space.

You are usually unaware of the space you occupy and how your movements take place within it. Because Pilates demands that you move and breathe correctly, you will become more aware, through concentration and the use of precision, of how your personal space is created. It is through precision that you can attain graceful movement.

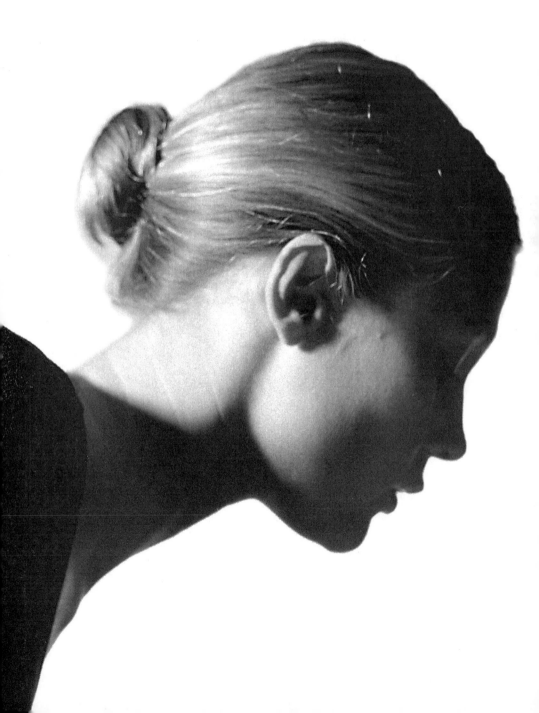

isolation

The Pilates technique is an excellent way of educating yourself and understanding, through movement, how your body works, in part and as a whole. Harmony comes from the integration of isolated parts.

"Each muscle may cooperatively and loyally aid in the uniform development of all our muscles." Joseph Pilates

For many years exercise teachers have talked about isolating different muscles. Yet it is only theoretically possible to see them in isolation; in practice, your muscles work together in groups. Often, in regular exercise classes focus has been on "spot reducing" certain areas to achieve a desired look. But in doing this you develop one muscle at the expense of another. Consequently, the whole balance of the body is thrown out of kilter. This "lopsided" approach is altogether at odds with the logic of the Pilates method.

Muscle balance

So, when we talk about isolation in Pilates we are simply making sure that you identify all your muscles for yourself, especially the weaker ones. Pilates exercises ensure you develop the neglected areas of the body that work alongside opposing, stronger muscles. For example, if you are a golfer, you know that when you play, you only stronger you will remain proportionally imbalanced.

Try the "Touch and visualize" exercise (see box) to better understand how your muscles work. Learn to identify the location of, say, your tricep without actually having to touch it. Visualization techniques help you connect mentally with the muscle. Over time you will be able to feel and identify various muscles working in combination as you perform the movements.

swing in one direction. Over a period of time your body then becomes over-trained in this direction. Although not all of us play golf, we all harbor muscle imbalances to some degree. It is not uncommon to discover these over- or under-trained areas through Pilates.

Weak links

Try to be aware of any imbalance in muscle strength or flexibility as you perform the movements. Your goal here is to work toward strengthening the weaker of the two sets of muscles so that balance is regained. Otherwise, as you get

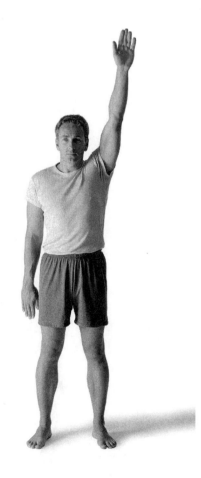

workout

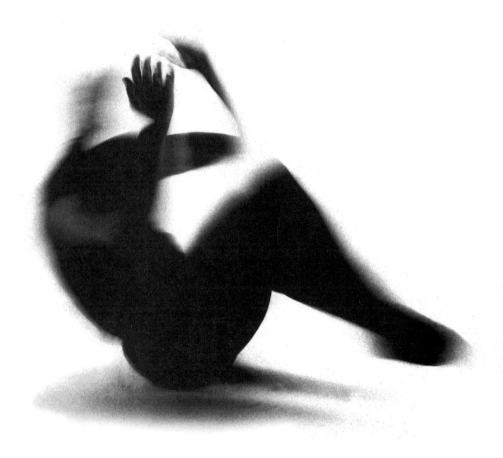

warm-ups

The warm-up exercises are designed to mobilize, lengthen, and stretch the muscles in preparation for more demanding movements. Use them to familiarize yourself with how your body feels as it moves and to focus on your breathing and posture before moving on to the main exercises.

one-arm circles

This movement opens up the shoulder joints.

▌ CAUTION

Do not lock your elbows and always work within your limits. If you find that you are able to make bigger circles on one side than the other, work on the weaker side in order to achieve balance in the body.

reps	10 times each side
visual cue	drawing circles
emphasis	mobility

1 Stand tall with your feet apart, knees soft. Reach up from the top of your head to the ceiling to check that your back is correctly aligned. Keeping your right arm by your side, pressed lightly against the leg, breathe in and lift your left arm in front of you and slightly to the side.

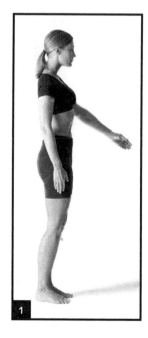

one-arm circles

2 Keeping the ribcage still, start to draw a circle with the arm as you breathe out. If the ribcage moves, you are swinging too far—move the arm farther away from the body to the side and draw a smaller circle. Imagine that you are drawing on the wall to the side of you with your fingertips.

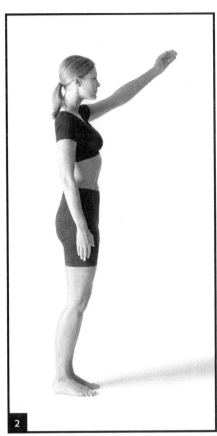

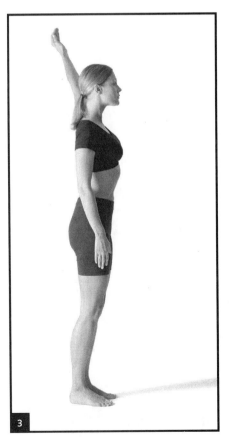

WORKOUT

3 Complete the circle, trying at all times to keep a slow, consistent speed. Imagine a wheel turning, with continuous motion and no sudden jolts. When you have completed 10 circles on one arm, change arms and repeat.

the cat

Imagine you are drawing up into yourself as you breathe out. Then, as you breathe in, gradually lengthen down and out of the position. Be sure the movements are continuous, that each flows smoothly into the next one.

reps	5–10 times
visual cue	a cat stretching
emphasis	mobility of the spine

1 From a standing position, bend your knees and place your hands just above them without applying undue pressure on the knee joint. Your back should be flat and in the neutral position, and your head and neck should be in line. Concentrate on a spot on the floor in front of you so that your head does not drop or look up. Breathe in to prepare for the next stage.

2 As you breathe out, draw up through the center of your back in the same way a cat does when it is stretching. Open your back as much as possible without losing the shape of the lower body. As you breathe in, lower the back down to the neutral position.

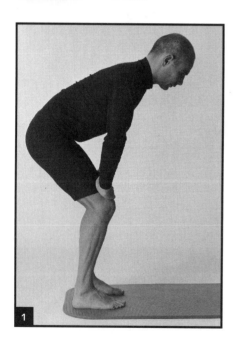

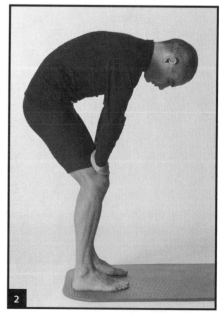

swinging

The swinging movement should feel continuous and flowing. Only go as low as you feel comfortable with: as your body becomes warmer, you may be able to move down a little lower.

reps	5–10 times
visual cue	rag doll
emphasis	strength

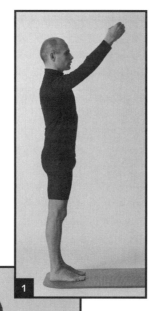

1 Stand tall in the neutral position. Then, with your eyes lifted, breathe in to prepare yourself and float your arms up in front of you without allowing your shoulder blades to lift.

2 Softly bend your knees, allow your arms to relax, then slowly move into a great downward scooping movement, breathing out as you go.

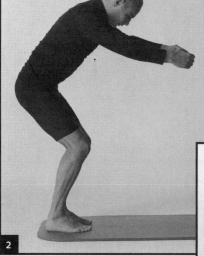

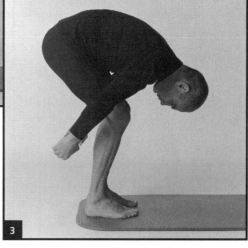

3 Continue with the movement while remembering to keep the knees soft. As you start to breathe in, slowly uncurl until you are upright again.

standing spine twist

Concentrate on lengthening and maintaining the third notch on the belt (see page 29). As you rotate, focus on keeping your hips facing forward with both feet planted on the ground, rather than allowing the hips to rotate with you.

reps	5–10 times each side
visual cue	corkscrew
emphasis	spine mobility

1 Standing tall in the neutral position, place the hands together in a praying gesture. Softly draw the shoulder blades back and then down into a soft "V." The thumbs should be placed on the sternum. Keep the thumbs there throughout the exercise so that the movement involves more than the arms. Take a breath in to prepare yourself.

2 As you breathe out, slowly rotate to the right, keeping the thumbs on the sternum and the nose in line with the thumbs. Focus on moving from the area between the shoulder blades. The whole center column should rotate as a single unit; don't let the head or arms rotate on their own. As you breathe in, rotate back to the center. On the next outbreath, rotate to the left, then back to the center as you breathe in. When rotating, allow your breathing rate to control the speed of the movement. Try to lengthen your spine a little farther each time you rotate back to the center.

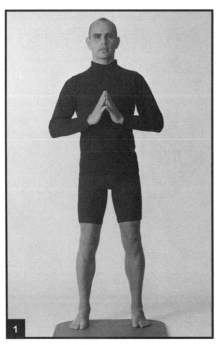

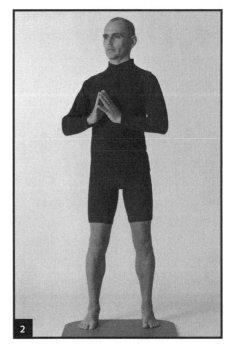

spine swing

Try not to overrotate the movement from the hips; instead, maintain the length in your lower spine. Keep the shoulders drawn down into the soft "V" and the belt muscle on the third notch (see page 29).

reps	5–10 times each side
visual cue	trailing hands
emphasis	spine mobility

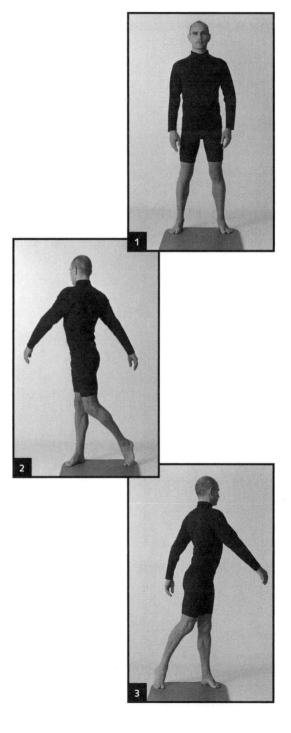

1 Stand tall with the spine in the neutral position and the feet slightly farther apart than the hips. Breathe in to prepare yourself.

2 As you breathe out, slowly rotate to the right, allowing the left heel to lift slightly. Keep the arms relaxed beside you and your knees soft and relaxed. Allow your head to turn to look over your shoulder.

3 Breathe in and rotate to the other side, keeping the movement continuously flowing with no breaks in the middle. The arms are relaxed and the heels lift naturally as you rotate.

balance 1

reps	5 times each side
visual cue	tightrope
emphasis	balance

1 Stand tall in the neutral position and keep your eyes focused on a point in front of you as if you are looking toward the horizon. Keep your hips as still as possible and lengthen out your right toe in front of you, keeping the toe in contact with the floor. The hips should be still, shoulder blades drawn down into a soft "V," and the arms relaxed beside you. The belt muscle should be on the third notch (see page 29).

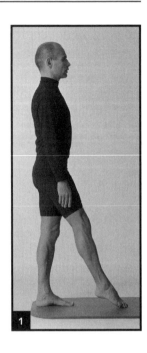

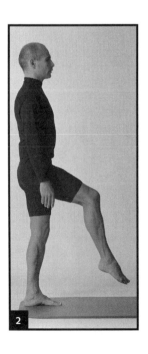

2 As you breathe out, slowly lift the right foot off the floor with the knee bent and the foot relaxed. Concentrate on keeping the left knee slightly bent, the hips still, and the weight even in the left foot. Imagine three points on the sole of your left foot: one under the big toe, one under the little toe, and one under the heel. Aim to keep an even pressure across all three points.

52

WORKOUT

balance 2

Keep the weight evenly distributed across the left foot in the same way as the previous balance exercise. Be sure that the supporting knee remains soft.

reps	5 times each side
visual cue	tightrope
emphasis	balance

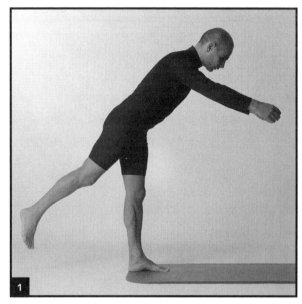

1 Starting from the neutral position, breathe out and lengthen the right leg and right arm. Don't lift the leg too high and lean slightly forward to allow the spine to remain lengthened and neutral. Keep the eyes looking down so that the neck stays in a neutral position.

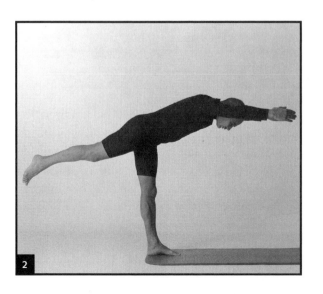

2 Keep lengthening through the movement until you reach a position where you feel you can maintain the balance and a neutral spine. Think about lengthening along the whole of the spine, from the head to the tailbone. As you breathe in, with control, reverse the movement to finish in a tall, standing position.

core elements

These are the building blocks of the Pilates technique. Take your time to work through each exercise. Listen to your body—you should never struggle to complete any of the movements.

the hundred

As you move your legs, brace your center to keep firm support. Keep both hips level as you lift your leg.

 CAUTION

Remain focused on keeping your body in the neutral position. Check that the size of the arch in your lower back has not increased or decreased as you lift and lower your leg.

reps	10 times
visual cue	steep slope
emphasis	abdominal strength

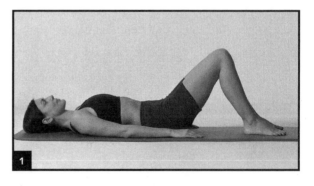

1 Lie on your back with your knees bent and your feet flat on the floor, comfortably close to your butt. Find the neutral position and, with your arms by your side, draw the shoulders back and down. Imagine that there is an orange between your chin and chest, and try to lengthen through the back of the neck.

the hundred

2 As you breathe out, lift the left leg to form a right angle, checking that the knee comes directly above the hip and that the foot is in line with the knee. Imprint your lower spine firmly into the mat.

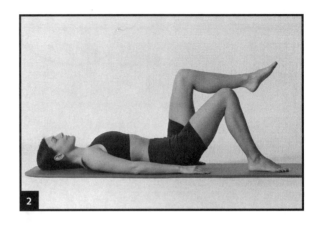

3 Lift the second leg and allow the spine to return to the neutral position.

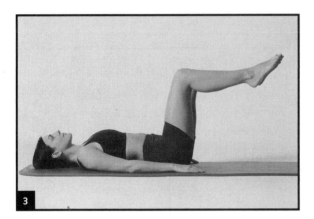

4 Lengthen your legs diagonally toward the ceiling. Hold for five breaths, focusing on not letting the abdominal muscles dome or the lower spine come out of the neutral position. On the last breath, lower one leg at a time, and return to the starting position.

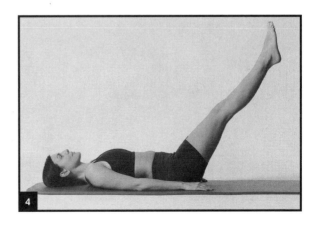

rocker with open legs

This movement works on the mobility of the spine. With the legs lifted you are also building up your strength.

reps	10 times
visual cue	rocking chair
emphasis	mobility

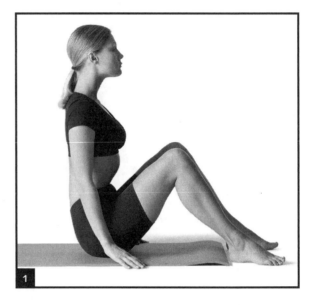

1 Sit with your legs in front of you, knees up and slightly apart. Lift up your head as though it is strung to the ceiling. Pull in your abs. Open your shoulders, rolling them well down your back.

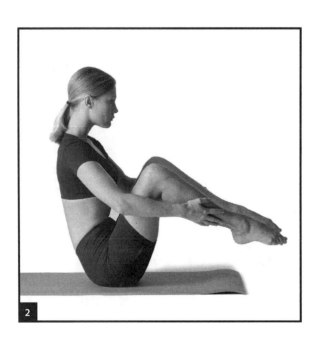

2 Hold your ankles and lift your legs to a balanced position. Push your legs away from you as you lift your head to maintain a long spine.

rocker with open legs

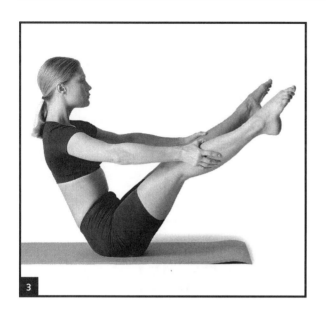

3 Keeping your balance, reach your legs out in front of you. The farther you extend your legs the more you need to pull in your abs to maintain balance.

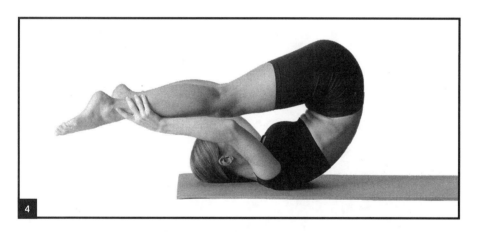

4 Breathe in as you roll back, keeping your legs the same distance from your body. Breathe out as you return to the balance position. Bend your knees slightly so you can touch your toes.

swimming

Imagine that a laser beam is being projected underneath you, following the direction of your spine between your arms and legs. You must avoid touching the beam. Soften the elbows and keep the hips stable.

▌CAUTION
■

Avoid locking the elbows and having the knees too close or too far apart.

reps	20 times each side
visual cue	glasses of water balanced on back
emphasis	strength

1 Kneel on the floor, lean forward, and place your hands under your shoulders. Your knees should be positioned below your hips, hip-width apart. Find your neutral spine position, keep your head level, and create a slight contraction of the center (see page 28). Avoid rounding the shoulders and keep your shoulder blades drawn down your back. The front of the chest should be kept "open," pushed forward proudly like a soldier on parade with the shoulder blades down and back. This creates a strong base or starting position.

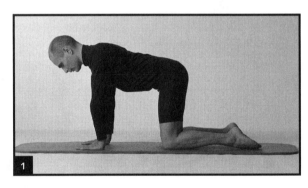

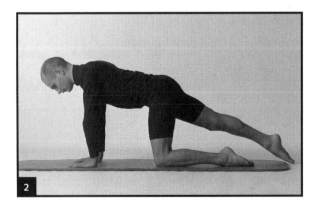

2 Focus on holding this position while you extend your right leg, toes pointed, behind you as you breathe out. Breathe in as you return to the starting position, placing the weight back on the knee. Repeat the movement with the left leg. The challenge is to prevent the movement and leg transition from affecting the stable position of the body.

58

WORKOUT

swimming

3 A different challenge is to start with the arms. In the same way as the leg exercise, reach out in front of you with alternate arms. Keep the fingers in contact with the floor and control the shoulder blades so that they stay down the back. Make an effort to keep the upper body in the neutral position and avoid taking all the weight on the knees. Imagine that your back is a tray with a full glass of water in each corner and you can't spill any water as you move.

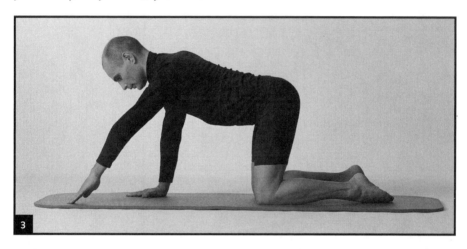

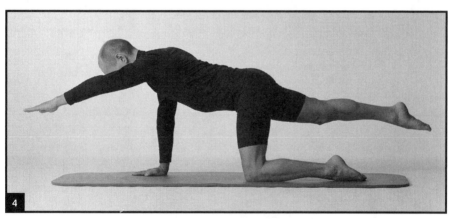

4 Once you have mastered this exercise, start extending your arms or your legs. At full reach, raise the arm or leg to shoulder or hip height. Only continue with this if you are able to maintain the slight contraction of the center. Finally, you can introduce balancing skills by lengthening the opposite arm and leg to create a diagonal across the body. The greatest challenge is on the transfer to the other side. Keep the arm and leg movement synchronized, lowering them before returning to the initial position.

push-up

reps	5–10 times
visual cue	snail on wall
emphasis	strength

1 Stand tall in the neutral position with feet hip-width apart and shoulders drawn back and down. Imagine your eyes are looking over the horizon, and take a breath in to prepare for the movement.

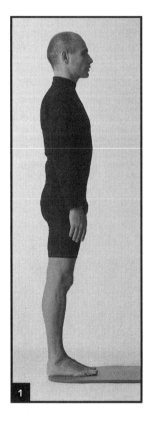

2 As you breathe out, begin to roll your head and spine downward, starting from the neck. Imagine each vertebra is in a chain that is moving link by link. Allow the weight of your arms to carry you forward.

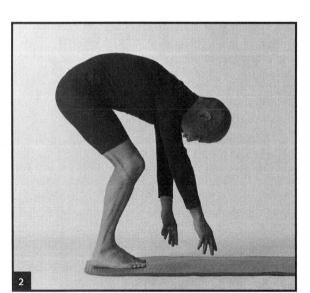

push-up

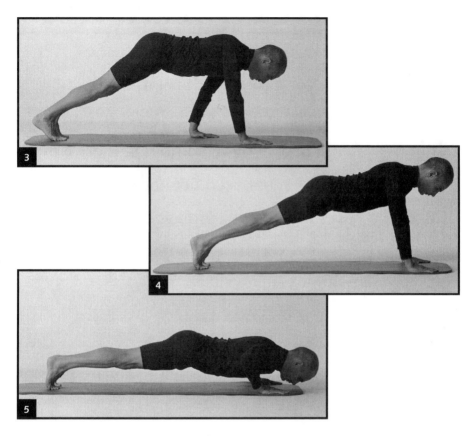

3 As you reach toward the floor, breathe in and bend your knees to enable your hands to touch the floor. As you breathe out, walk your hands along the floor. Keep your back level and think about keeping your butt in line with your shoulders.

4 Before moving to the push-up phase of this movement, check that your body is in correct alignment to avoid straining your joints. Your hands should be directly under the shoulders, your shoulders drawn back and down away from the ears, your neck relaxed, and your eyes looking toward the floor.

5 Keeping alignment neutral, inhale and lower your body toward the floor. Draw the shoulders back and down as you do so, trying to keep the back neutral and your butt in line with your shoulders. Go as low as you can without losing the correct body alignment. Work back slowly through the positions until you return to the standing position.

powerhouse abs

As you progress through this section, which focuses on the lower half of the body, you will find that these movements become more difficult. It's fine to challenge yourself but don't exceed the comfortable range of movement.

neck pull

This movement builds strength and tests your ability to lift the body from the floor.

reps	10 times
visual cue	folding over
emphasis	strength

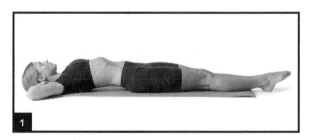

1

1 Lie on the floor with your arms behind your head and your fingers clasped. Stretch your legs out straight with your toes pointing away from you. Check that your back is in neutral position and you are pulling in on your center.

neck pull

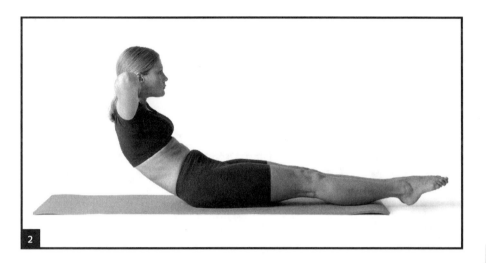

2 Slowly roll forward and peel your back off the floor as you breathe out. Keep the movement very smooth and slow. (If you feel any strain in your back let your arms down. Pull in and up on your abs and bend your knees.)

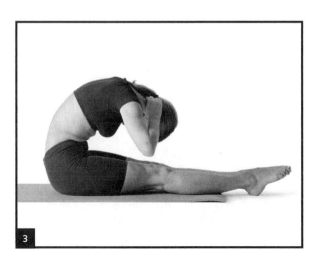

3 Stretch forward to the point of tension and then, without stopping, roll back down, laying your vertebrae onto the mat one by one. Try to be aware of each disc and feel each vertebra imprint into your mat, imagining that the mat is made out of soft putty.

single-leg stretch

Focus on stabilizing the hips and maintaining neutral as you lengthen the leg. Your shoulder blades should remain drawn back and down.

▌ CAUTION

Make sure that the arch in the lower back does not increase or decrease as you lift and lower the legs.

reps	5–10 times each side
visual cue	toe reach
emphasis	strength

1 Lie on your back with your knees bent and your feet flat on the floor comfortably close to your butt. Find neutral and, with your arms by your sides, draw the shoulders back and down. Imagine an orange between your chin and chest, and try to lengthen through the back of the neck.

2 As you breathe out, lift the left leg to a right angle. Check that the knee is directly above the hip and that the foot is in line with the knee. As you hold this position, focus on keeping the hips still and braced.

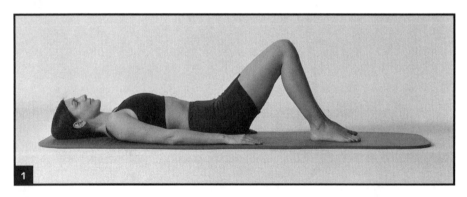

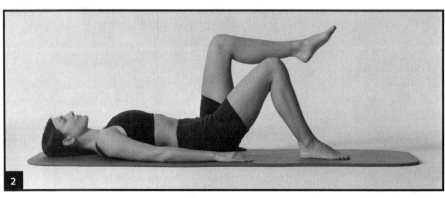

single-leg stretch

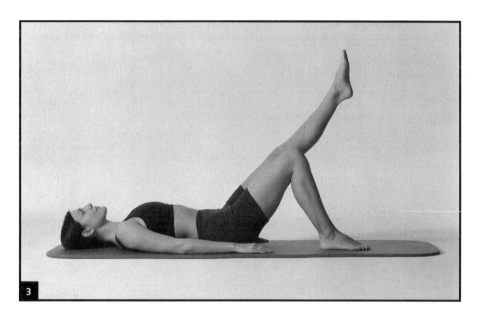

3 Keep your arms relaxed beside you; while you can use them for some support, avoid gripping the floor with them. As you breathe out, lengthen the left leg diagonal toward the ceiling. Concentrate on maintaining neutral and keeping the hips braced.

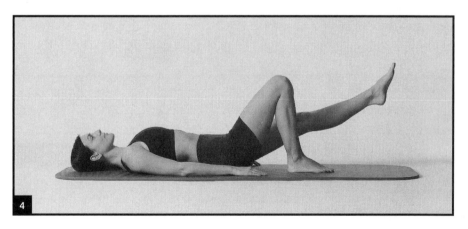

4 Lower the leg toward the floor—the lower the leg, the greater the challenge is to maintain the neutral position. As you breathe in, return the leg to a right-angle position. Lengthen the leg five times, then slowly return it back to the starting position.

leg pull prone

Joseph Pilates was inspired by yoga, and this movement is very similar to the plank position. With Pilates, the focus is on the movement as you pass through the plank position.

▌ CAUTION

If your breathing gets faster you are working too hard. Progress is achieved by taking it slowly.

reps	10 times
visual cue	coffee table
emphasis	strength

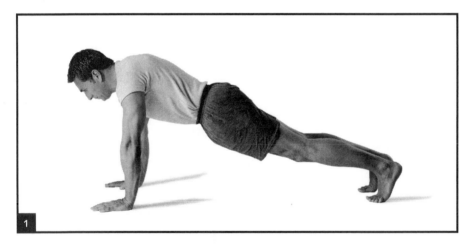

1

1 Start in a push-up position with your back in a straight line and your abs tucked in to protect your back. Be sure not to let your butt lift higher than your shoulders. Keep your shoulders pulled down and held in place; do not lock your elbows. Breathe in.

leg pull prone

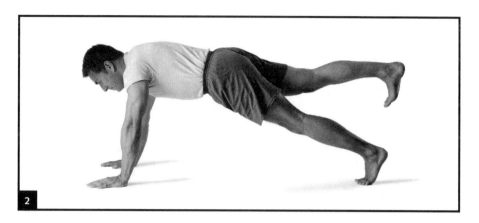

2 Breathe out as you raise your right leg, not letting your hips move. Initiate the lift by contracting your abs. Pretend you are a puppet: when you pull the string of the puppet the leg lifts. Your string is your abs being tightened.

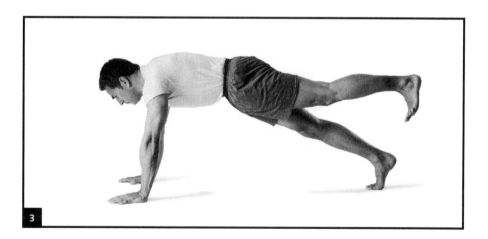

3 Breathe in as you lower the leg and breathe out as you change to lift up the other leg. Your goal should be to make sure that your hips do not move. Keep your back straight. Check that your shoulder blades are pulled down your back and that your neck is stretched. Legs should be lifted and lowered slowly and continuously, with no change in speed.

up a tree

Try to keep the knees as straight as possible without locking the knee joint. This will ensure that the stretch also runs up through the back of the knee.

reps	5–10 times each side
visual cue	climbing
emphasis	abdominal strength

WORKOUT

1 Lie on your back with your legs straight, and find the neutral spine position. On your next outbreath, raise your right leg toward the ceiling and place your hands on the back of your right thigh. Try to keep your leg as straight as possible, without locking your knee. Keep your shoulders drawn back and down and your neck relaxed.

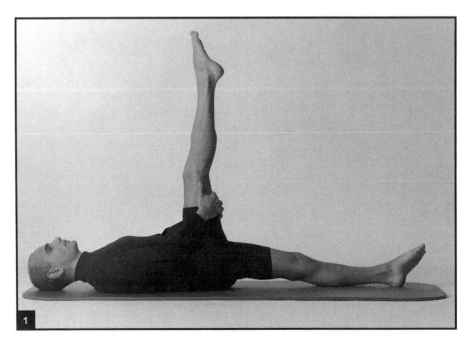

1

up a tree

2 On the next outbreath, start to walk your hands one over the other as you climb toward your foot: your head and shoulders will lift off the floor as you proceed. As you walk your hands up your leg, imagine that you are climbing up a tree.

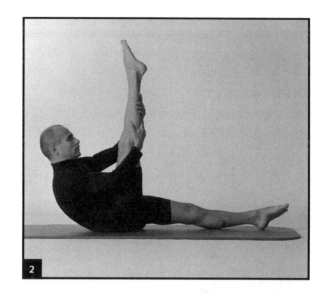

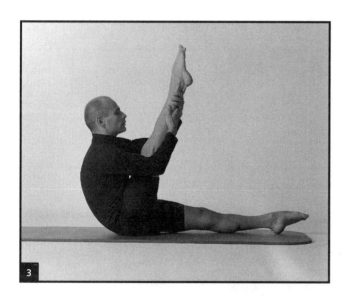

3 Keep climbing your hands up your leg until you have gone as far as possible without overstraining. Take a breath in and as you breathe out, reverse the whole exercise, walking your hands down until your head and shoulders are back on the floor.

leg pull supine

This movement builds strength as you test your abs to keep your hips aloft while you move your legs.

▮ CAUTION

Keep your body weight off your shoulders by pulling your shoulder blades down your back and keeping your neck stretched long.

reps	5–10 times
visual cue	scissors
emphasis	leg and abdominal strength

1 Start in a sitting position with your legs straight in front of you. Place your hands on the floor, shoulder-width apart, with your fingers pointing toward your knees. Keep the top of your head lifted up toward the ceiling. Pull your abs in and pull your shoulder blades down your back.

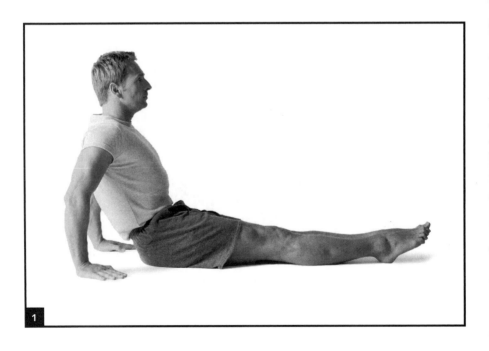

1

leg pull supine

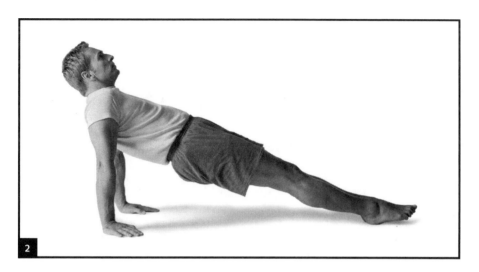

2

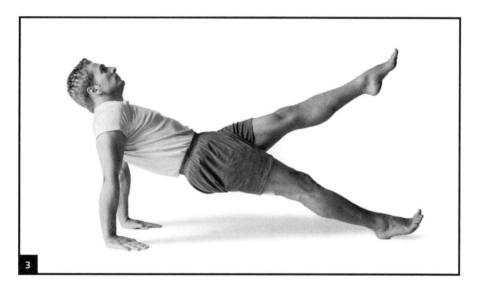

3

2 Breathe in as you raise your hips to the ceiling, making a straight line from your shoulders through your hips and ankles.

3 Breathe out as you raise your left leg to the ceiling, keeping your hips in a fixed position. Focus on your center of power to lift your legs. Breathe in as you lower one leg and change to the other. Repeat 10 times on each leg before slowly lowering it. Keep the flow continuous as you change legs.

the jack knife

This is a strength maneuver that challenges you to lift the body up into a shoulder stand.

 CAUTION

Check that you have enough flexibility in the spine before you try this. By bending your knees during the movement you can reduce stress on the lower back.

reps	10 times
visual cue	jack knife
emphasis	strength

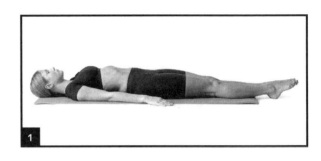

1 Lie flat on the floor with your arms down by your side. Stretch your head away from you.

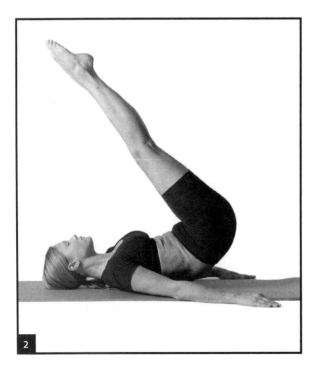

2 Breathe out and lift your legs slowly up to the ceiling. Keep your feet above your face as they stretch upward. Try not to use your arms too much: use your center as a powerhouse.

the jack knife

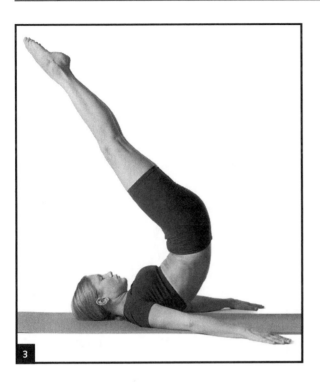

3 When you reach the highest point of your leg roll, hold for two breaths.

4 On the second outbreath, slowly let your body down. It is not the stretch at the top of the movement that should be your goal but rather the journey getting there and coming back.

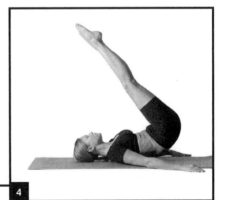

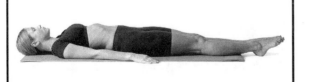

5 Return to the starting position. The slower you do this movement, the more you will develop your strength.

swan dive

This is an advanced move, so progress to this only when you have worked with the other exercises shown here for six months.

reps	5–10 times
visual cue	rocking horse
emphasis	spine and abdomen strength and mobility

1 Starting from the facedown position, place your arms, palms in, by your sides. Draw your shoulder blades back and down.

2 Breathing out slowly, float your chest away from the floor. As you breathe in, lower it again. Lift with the muscles of the back in the thoracic area. As you lift, lengthen the muscles in the lower part of the spine. If the muscles in the lower back tighten or pinch, relax down and rest.

WORKOUT

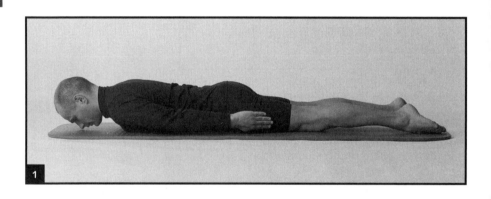

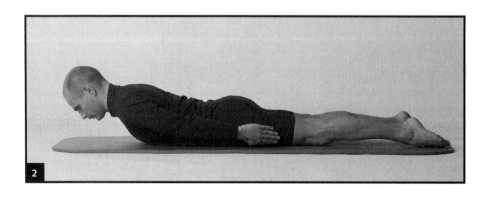

advanced swan dive

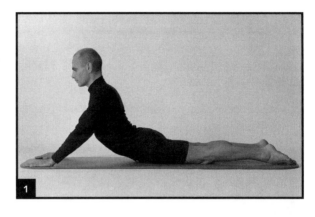

1 Lying on your front, extend your arms in front of you in the cobra position. Try not to compress the lower spine. Lift from the lower abdominals and hips instead. Breathe in to lift.

75

WORKOUT

2 As you breathe out, allow your body weight to tip forward onto your chest and your legs to lift behind you just like a counterbalance.

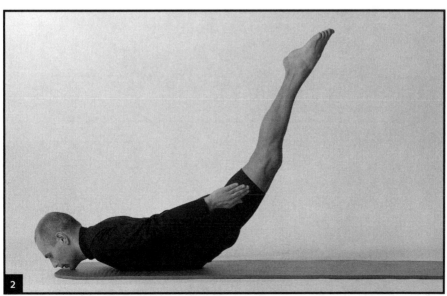

roll-up

Imagine that your spine is a chain or a system of links: each area of the spine should work independently as you work through the movement to create a smooth, chain-like movement.

█ CAUTION

Keep your feet on the floor, and avoid spurts of speed as you roll up: the move should be smooth and continuous.

reps	5–10 times
visual cue	the morning sun rising
emphasis	abdominal strength

1 Lie on your back with your legs straight and your arms stretched over your head. Draw your shoulder blades back and down.

2 As you breathe out, begin to peel your head and shoulders off the floor, and slowly lift your arms toward the ceiling as you come up.

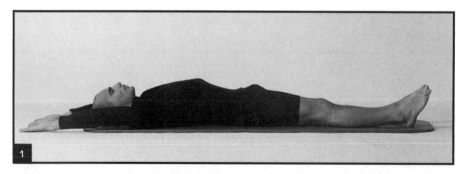

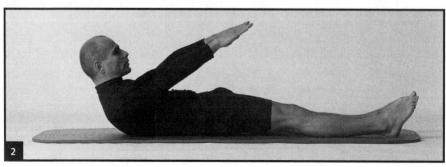

roll-up

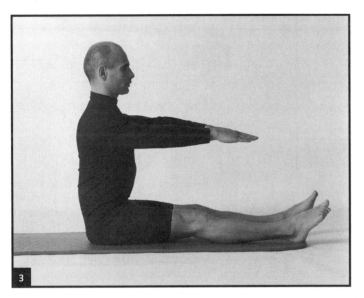

3 Continue to roll forward slowly, peeling your spine off the floor vertebra by vertebra. Roll through the pelvis until you reach a sitting position.

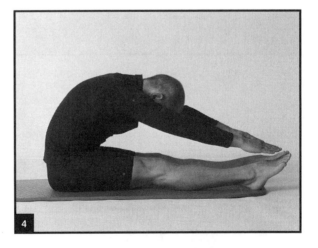

4 Breathe in as you lengthen out over your legs, stretching your arms toward your toes as far as you feel comfortable. As you breathe out, reverse the move and slowly lower your body back onto the mat: begin by rolling through the pelvis, then roll down vertebra by vertebra.

the teaser

This movement is designed to increase strength. You challenge the body by lifting the torso up to a balanced position.

▮ CAUTION

The degree of intensity entailed in this movement can be decreased by keeping one leg on the floor at all times.

reps	10 times
visual cue	horizontal dive
emphasis	strength

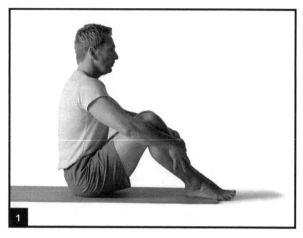

1 Sit with your knees bent in front of you and hold your legs lightly. Pull up on your center as you straighten your head and pull yourself up toward the ceiling.

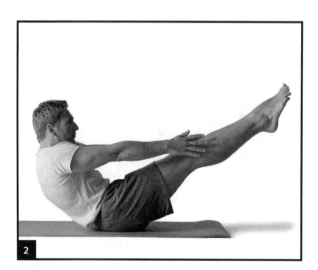

2 Breathe in and extend your legs, keeping a balanced position. Slowly lift your hands up toward your feet. Remember to keep your shoulder blades down your back.

the teaser

3 Feel your spine lifting off the mat, vertebra by vertebra. See how far you can extend yourself before you lose control of the movement.

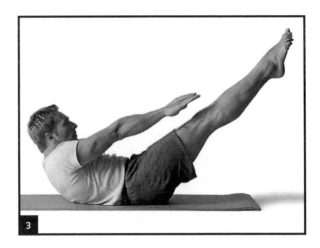

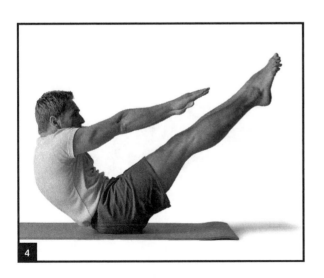

4 Breathe in as you let your body slowly roll down to the mat, and breathe out as you come back up to the balanced position. Keep the movement slow and smooth as you repeat it 10 times.

side bend

This movement builds strength as it challenges you to lift your body weight off the floor.

▋ CAUTION

Pressure against a joint is good because it squeezes out all the old synovial fluid and draws in new fluid. But if you feel pressure at your elbow or wrist, stop.

reps	10 times each side
visual cue	leaning tower
emphasis	strength

1 Sit on your right hip with your right arm straight, your hand below your shoulder. Bend your left leg and place it in front of your right leg, which should be straight. Lift your head and tuck in your abs. Try to keep your hips forward so they are stacked one on top of the other.

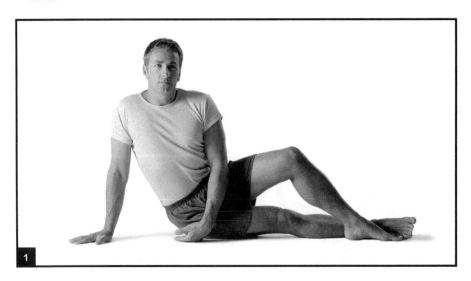

1

side bend

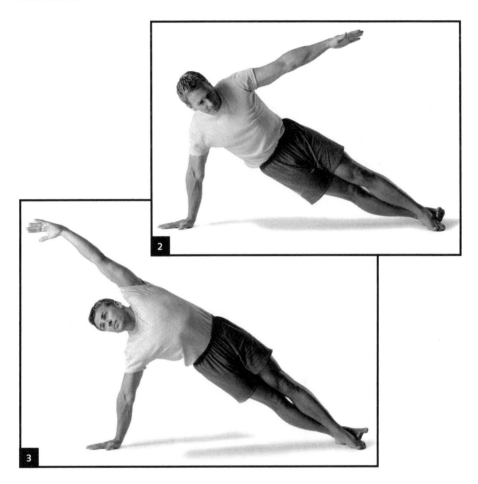

2 Breathe out as you push on your left foot and start lifting your body toward the ceiling. Reach out and up to the ceiling as your left arm draws a semicircle through the air along your side. Your strength is in your center, which pulls in to create the movement. Keep your spine long as you begin to lift.

3 Continue to stretch until you are fully extended. Breathe in as you slowly lower your body back to the starting position. Keep your speed the same when you move up and when you come down. Try to support yourself and keep your weight steady between each movement until you have completed the 10 repetitions.

scissors

This is a strength movement that challenges you to stay balanced as you change legs.

▌ CAUTION

Don't let your leg drop toward you. It will help if you keep focused on the leg that is the farthest away from your trunk. Let this leg lead the slow "snipping" move.

WORKOUT

reps	10 times
visual cue	scissors
emphasis	strength

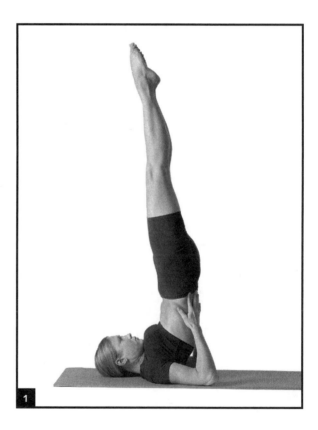

1 Lie on the floor, arms by your sides. Breathe out as you lift your body into a shoulder-stand position using the movement of a jack knife (page 72). Place your hands behind your back for support.

scissors

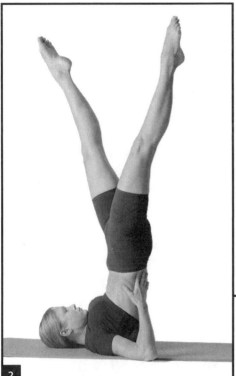

2 Breathe out as you open your legs an equal distance apart. Point your feet to the ceiling, stretching them as far as you can to lengthen the legs.

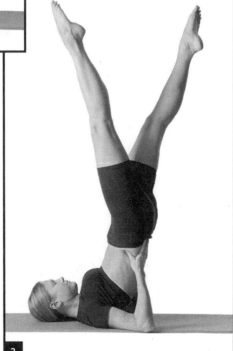

3 Breathe in as they close and change to the other side. Keep the movement consistent and slow as you find out how wide you can make each "snipping" move without your hips moving. Keep your hips pointing to the ceiling by using your abs to lift their weight off your elbows. Lengthen your neck and keep your shoulder blades pulled up, not crunched up.

shoulder bridge

84

This movement tests your core strength.

! CAUTION

Don't arch your back too far. Keep your shoulders, hips, and knees in a straight line.

reps	10 times each side
visual cue	ship's mast
emphasis	strength

1 Lie on your back with your knees bent and feet hip-width apart. Stretch your arms down by your side and stretch your spine up toward your head.

2 Breathe in as you roll your hips up toward the ceiling, peeling your spine from the mat vertebra by vertebra. Keep your abs pulled in. Only roll up as far as your shoulders.

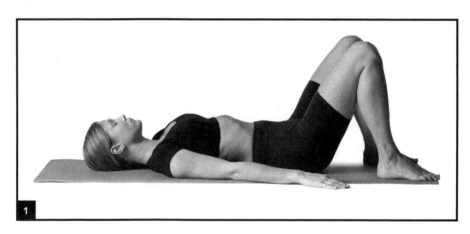

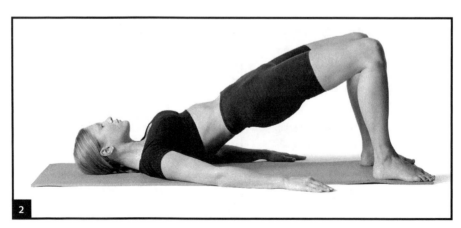

shoulder bridge

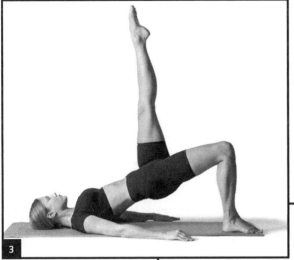

3 Breathe out as you unfold your left leg up toward the ceiling, keeping your hips at the same height and not allowing them to drop. Use the strength in your center to hold you in place.

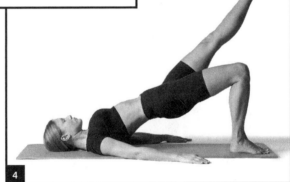

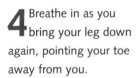

4 Breathe in as you bring your leg down again, pointing your toe away from you.

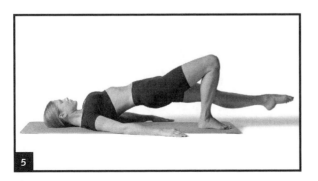

5 Try to touch the floor as you stretch the leg down. Breathe out as you lift the leg back to the ceiling. Breathe in as you touch the floor again. Slowly breathe out as you roll the spine back down, laying the vertebrae back onto the mat one by one.

the corkscrew

This movement builds strength and demands that you control the move even as you spin off balance.

▌ CAUTION

It is very important that before you challenge yourself with an off-balance move you have built up enough strength at your center.

reps	10 times
visual cue	side twist
emphasis	strength

WORKOUT

1 Lie flat on the floor with your arms by your sides. Breathe out as you slowly raise your legs and torso up and over your head, letting your toes touch the floor. Slowly peel your back off the floor. Keep your arms down by your side to help you up off the floor; check that your shoulder blades are pulled down your back. Breathe in when you reach the top point of the movement.

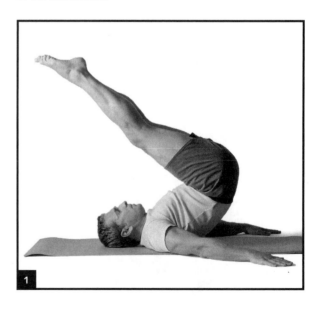

the corkscrew

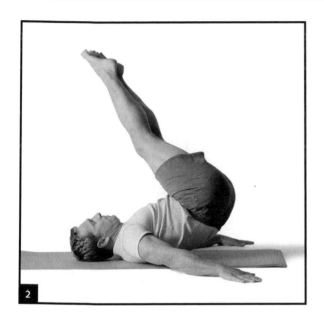

2 Breathe out and let your legs start drawing a semicircle together. Start with a small circle to keep control, then try to find the point where you threaten to lose control. Feel the one side of your spine laying down on the floor as you complete the semicircle.

WORKOUT

3 As your tailbone touches the floor slowly breathe in and repeat the movement, lifting your legs up and over your head. This time, take the semicircle to the other side. Work evenly on each side and remember—the slower the movement, especially on the downward phase, the more strength you are building. Keep your actions continuous, flowing evenly.

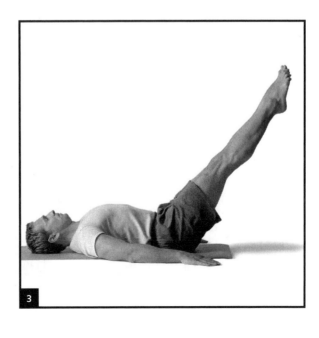

rolling–teaser–jack knife

For more details on the jack knife and the teaser, see page 72 and page 78 respectively. Try to link the movements together. Listen to your body. If you become tired, stop or lower the level of intensity.

WORKOUT

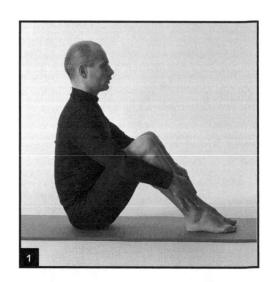

1 Start in a seated position with your hands clasped around your ankles.

2 As you begin to roll up out of the seated position, hold in a balance position and extend your legs into the teaser. Place your hands beside you to find a balance position without losing neutral spine.

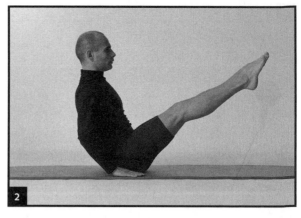

3 Once you feel confident, take your hands away and, keeping them at shoulder height, reach toward your feet. As you breathe out, lengthen your chest toward your feet.

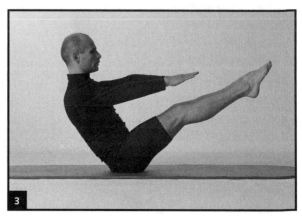

rolling–teaser–jack knife

4 Slowly lower your head and shoulders to the floor while keeping your legs lifted in a diagonal position as you breathe out.

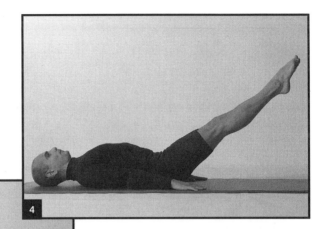

5 Begin to peel the lower part of your spine off the floor. As you peel the spine off the floor, your legs will begin to lift over your head. Continue to peel the spine off the floor until you are resting on your shoulders and your legs are lengthened toward the ceiling.

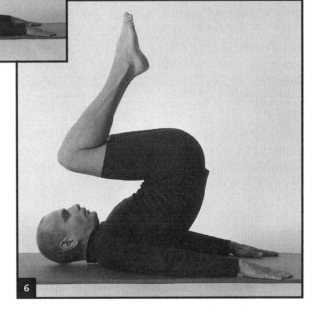

6 Hold for two breaths. On your second outbreath, draw your knees toward your chest. Then complete the rolling until you are back to sitting up in the starting position.

glossary

Abdominal muscles (abs): the muscles layered across the midriff that lie across each other at various angles. There are four types: the rectus abdominals, internal obliques, external obliques, and transversus abdominals.

Aerobic exercise: any sustained activity that works the heart and lungs, increasing the amount of oxygen in the blood.

Alignment: arrangement in a straight line.

Cardiovascular: relating to the heart or the blood vessels.

Centering movements: the Pilates exercises that work the center of the body, abdominals, and back.

Core exercises: the Pilates movements that concentrate on strengthening the abdominal and back muscles.

Crunching: sit-ups where the abdominals are not engaged so much as squeezed together, shortening the space between the hips and ribcage.

C-shape: the shape of the spine when the body is slumped over and bent due to bad posture.

Elongation: lengthening of the muscle. Leaner muscles develop from stretching the muscle rather than bulking it up.

Hidden stress: when muscle groups compensate for an injury or difficulty by using larger muscles to protect weaker ones.

Hyperextension: extending further than 180 degrees. Hyperextension occurs when the muscles tense up and the elbows or knees lock, resulting in a reverse bending.

Imprinting: gently pushing each vertebra into the mat, as though it were leaving an indentation.

Lumbar curve: the bend of the spine at the small of the back.

Neutral spine: the spine in its most natural position, which might not necessarily feel comfortable or "normal."

Overloading: point where the effort required by a muscle to withstand an applied weight is too great. The tissue may tear or rupture as a result.

Powerhouse: the name that Joseph Pilates gave to the abdominal area, found between our ribcage and hips.

Pilates exercises work this area in order to create a stronger, more balanced lower back.

Prone: lying facedown.

Resistance: an opposing force that pulls in the direction opposite to the one created by your muscle.

Rolling: exercises where the spine rolls over the mat, one vertebra at a time.

Soft knees: holding the knees relaxed and slightly bent, rather than locked.

Supine: lying down on the back.

Tendon: elastic linking tissue that connects bone to muscle.

Tripod position: where the feet support the body weight by distributing it evenly over three points: the ball of the foot, the middle of the heel, and the outside edge of the foot, near the little toe.

Vertebra: one of the bony segments that make up the spinal column.

Visualization: use of mental imagery to aid the accomplishment of physical tasks—an important element of the Pilates technique that helps the mind more effectively control the body.

index

other Ulysses books

ASHTANGA YOGA FOR WOMEN:
INVIGORATING MIND, BODY, AND SPIRIT WITH POWER YOGA
Sally Griffyn, $17.95

Presents the exciting and empowering practice of power yoga in a balanced fashion that addresses the specific needs of female practitioners.

HOW TO MEDITATE: AN ILLUSTRATED GUIDE
TO CALMING THE MIND AND RELAXING THE BODY
Paul Roland, $16.95

Offers a friendly approach to calming the mind and raising consciousness through various techniques, including meditation, visualization, body scanning for tension, and mantras.

THE JOSEPH H. PILATES METHOD AT HOME:
A BALANCE, SHAPE, STRENGTH & FITNESS PROGRAM
Eleanor McKenzie, $16.95

This handbook describes and details Pilates, a mental and physical program that combines elements of yoga and classical dance.

PILATES PERSONAL TRAINER BACK STRENGTHENING WORKOUT:
ILLUSTRATED STEP-BY-STEP MATWORK ROUTINE
Michael King and Yolande Green, $9.95

The easy starter program in this workbook teaches Pilates exercises that are appropriate for strengthening the back in a safe and healthy manner.

PILATES PERSONAL TRAINER GETTING STARTED WITH STRETCHING:
ILLUSTRATED STEP-BY-STEP MATWORK ROUTINE
Michael King and Yolande Green, $9.95

Ideal for beginners or older people, the specially designed Pilates exercises in this book offer a gentle workout of light strength movements and key stretches.

PILATES PERSONAL TRAINER THIGHS & BUTT WORKOUT:
ILLUSTRATED STEP-BY-STEP MATWORK ROUTINE
Michael King and Yolande Green, $9.95

Instead of paying $100-plus per hour for private Pilates sessions, those looking to get the same kind of targeted workout to shape and slim their thighs and buttocks can find it in this book.

PILATES WORKBOOK:
ILLUSTRATED STEP-BY-STEP GUIDE TO MATWORK TECHNIQUES
Michael King, $12.95

Illustrates the core matwork movements exactly as Joseph Pilates intended them to be performed; readers learn each movement by following the photographic sequences and explanatory captions.

PILATES WORKBOOK FOR PREGNANCY:
ILLUSTRATED STEP-BY-STEP MATWORK TECHNIQUES
Michael King and Yolande Green, $12.95

Presented in an easy-to-use style with step-by-step photo sequences of Pilates matwork techniques—adapted here for pregnancy and post-pregnancy.

SENSES WIDE OPEN: THE ART & PRACTICE OF LIVING IN YOUR BODY
Johanna Putnoi, $14.95

Through simple, accessible exercises, this book shows how to be at ease with yourself and experience genuine pleasure in your physical connection to others and the world.

YOGA IN FOCUS: POSTURES, SEQUENCES, AND MEDITATIONS
Jessie Chapman   photographs by Dhyan, $14.95

A beautiful celebration of yoga that's both useful for learning the techniques and inspiring in its artistic approach to presenting the body in yoga positions.

YOGA FOR PARTNERS: OVER 75 POSTURES TO DO TOGETHER
Jessie Chapman   photographs by Dhyan, $14.95

An excellent tool for learning two-person yoga, *Yoga for Partners* features inspiring photos of the paired asanas. It teaches each partner how to synchronize their movements and breathing, bringing new lightness and enjoyment to any yoga practice.

OTHER ULYSSES BOOKS

To order these books call 800-377-2542 or 510-601-8301, fax 510-601-8307, e-mail ulysses@ulyssespress.com, or write to Ulysses Press, P.O. Box 3440, Berkeley, CA 94703. All retail orders are shipped free of charge. California residents must include sales tax. Allow two to three weeks for delivery.

about the authors

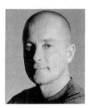

With more than two decades of experience in Pilates, **Michael King** first started working with the Pilates technique while he was a dancer at the London School of Contemporary Dance. He trained with Alan Herdman, the first teacher to bring Pilates to the United Kingdom from the United States. In 1982, he opened his own studio in London. Two years later, Michael moved to Texas, running a studio for the Houston Ballet Company while training in the new Fonda-established aerobics. Michael is the company director of the Pilates Institute, the United Kingdom's leading Pilates training company.

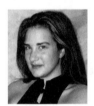

Yolande Green has been an instructor in the fitness industry for more than a decade, teaching aerobics, step, spinning, body conditioning, and Pilates. She is currently studying for an M.Sc. in health and fitness. Yolande is the company director of the Schools' Fitness Advisory Service, a training company for exercise teachers in secondary schools, and also serves as a presenter and tutor for the Pilates Institute. She has run many successful exercise and education groups, and has given presentations at fitness conventions and workshops around the world.

acknowledgments

Many thanks to all the instructors and staff at the Pilates Institute, not only in London but also in the many other countries that continue to promote the work of Joseph Pilates through our name. This book is dedicated to our great friend and colleague Sarah Irwin, who continues to be a great inspiration to many Pilates Instructors both here in the U.K. and in the U.S. where she lives.
—Michael King

I hope that this book enables people to learn and utilize the Pilates technique in the same way that I have. I would like to thank Michael for his time and mentoring and to acknowledge the support received from my Mum and Dad and my boyfriend Pete.
—Yolande Green